THE DOULAS

RADICAL CARE FOR PREGNANT PEOPLE

BY MARY MAHONEY &
LAUREN MITCHELL

FOREWORD BY LORETTA ROSS
AFTERWORD BY DR. WILLIE PARKER

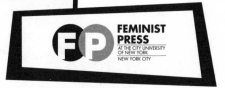

FEMINIST
PRESS
AT THE CITY UNIVERSITY
OF NEW YORK
NEW YORK CITY

Published in 2016 by the Feminist Press
at the City University of New York
The Graduate Center
365 Fifth Avenue, Suite 5406
New York, NY 10016

feministpress.org

First Feminist Press edition 2016

This book was made possible thanks to a grant from New York State Council
on the Arts with the support of Governor Andrew Cuomo and the New York
State Legislature.

First printing November 2016

Cover design and text design by Suki Boynton

Library of Congress Cataloging-in-Publication Data
Names: Mahoney, Mary, author. | Mitchell, Lauren.
Title: The Doulas : radical care for pregnant people / by Mary Mahoney and
  Lauren Mitchell.
Description: New York : The Feminist Press, 2016.
Identifiers: LCCN 2016015027 (print) | LCCN 2016026774 (ebook) | ISBN
  9781558619418 (paperback) | ISBN 9781558619494 (e-book)
Subjects: LCSH: Doulas. | Pregnancy. | Natural childbirth--Coaching. | BISAC:
  SOCIAL SCIENCE / Feminism & Feminist Theory. | MEDICAL / Nursing /
  Maternity, Perinatal, Women's Health. | HEALTH & FITNESS / Pregnancy &
  Childbirth. | SOCIAL SCIENCE / Women's Studies.
Classification: LCC RG950 .M33 2016 (print) | LCC RG950 (ebook) | DDC
  618.4/5--dc23
LC record available at https://lccn.loc.gov/2016015027

Like water on stone, I have loved them,
and they have marked me.

—NAOMI WALLACE, *One Flea Spare*

Contents

THE DOULAS

Thank God for the Doulas!

Most people have never heard of doulas, but I'd venture that all pregnant people could use one. Having a person who unconditionally nurtures you during a major life experience is a privilege too few enjoy. Doulas provide this exquisite nonjudgmental support to others—often strangers—and touch peoples' lives in profound ways.

The original doula was a female slave (from the Greek word "*doulē*"), and the term eventually evolved in the past forty or so years to designate women trained as birth attendants. In 2008, though, a trio of young activists launched the concept of "abortion doulas" into the zeitgeist. By imagining the doula role anew, they expanded the meaning of the word to include the full spectrum of possible pregnancy outcomes—births, adoptions, abortions, miscarriages, and deaths—as well as services to women, men, transgender, and gender nonconforming people.

These new doulas proudly bear witness to the lives of those they serve, transforming themselves in the process. With little experience but plenty of empathy, Lauren Mitchell and Mary Mahoney helped create a full-spectrum doula movement to expand the caregiving model into one that covers the entire range of life possibilities. As activists as well as service providers, they articulated a new dimension of the human rights movement for reproductive self-determination, based on passion, service, and advocacy.

An inspiring group of full-spectrum doulas tell their stories in this book. Some serve in hospitals. Others labor in abortion clinics or at adoption agencies. Others work in homes. Together, they represent a fresh generation of caregivers who weave diverse pregnancy experiences into a holistic service and advocacy model that challenges stigmatized, artificial divisions among pregnancy outcomes. The same people who give birth sometimes have abortions or miscarriages. Some births culminate in an adoption. Every pregnancy is different, and each has its own finale.

That simple truth is why this book is precious. The stories of these full-spectrum doulas and their collective knowledge help end the painful social stereotypes that cause pregnant people to be categorized as good or bad based on a pregnancy's outcome. Through the eyes of doulas, we witness the range of pregnancy experiences affected by imbalances of power, privilege, and knowledge, whether pregnant for four weeks or nine months. These doulas call it "story-based care" because they hear many stories of people for whom some choices are straightforward, while others offer extreme complexity, requiring the deftly engaged services of doulas who can handle both emotional and technical difficulties.

We also learn how important it is for doulas to take care of themselves in order to be brave for people whose experiences may be shrouded in stigma and secrecy. Doulas give so much emotional, physical, and spiritual support to others that they may fail to save some love for themselves. They join the movement to serve, not to be served. Because they see the macro-level systems that shape the experiences of their clients, they can let their desire to help fight injustices disguise their need to replenish themselves. But an empty vessel can't fill others. When they come up against burnout, cynicism, and rage, this new cadre of reproductive justice activists must help each other recalibrate, regroup, and reaffirm their commitment to themselves and others.

Unlike most caregiving services, abortion doulas are exposed to the physical and emotional dangers also faced by clinic doctors, nurses, receptionists, and escorts, some of whom have been killed or assaulted by violent vigilantes. After all, clinic escort James Barrett was killed in Pensacola, Florida, in 1994 along with the doctor, John Britton. In 2015 two civilians killed at a Colorado Springs Planned Parenthood—Jennifer Markovsky and Ke'Arre M. Stewart—were at the clinic supporting friends. Worrying about domestic terrorism while providing a medical service should not be a part of a doula's repertoire, but these activists generously help others navigate these perils, even as they face the threats themselves.

Like many, I experienced pregnancy as a totally life-altering event for which I was not prepared. I felt a confused mixture of wonder and terror during my first pregnancy as a teenager in the 1960s, not quite believing it was happening to me. I knew little about sex and less about pregnancy. I marveled at the changes in my body and its potential for motherhood. I felt like an adult emancipating from childhood. At the same time, I was in an exhausting state of denial. I remember hoping that the pregnancy would be gone when I woke up and my body would revert back to its prepregnancy state. Now, looking back as a grandmother, I know fear filled me. The primal fight or flight reflexes were dominant. And, because abortion was not legal at the time, my family knew of only two options for me: to keep the baby or choose adoption.

Full-spectrum doulas did not exist then, but I can tell you now that I desperately needed one. My mother was traumatized by the incest that led to my pregnancy and she scarcely knew how to advise me, much less offer any support or care. My father was angry that this had happened to his daughter, and felt powerless to visit his hurt and rage on our miscreant relative. While I was assured of their love, I didn't know anything about the process of pregnancy and birthing, or how to evaluate my few reproductive options.

My parents placed me in a Salvation Army home for unwed mothers, a barbed-wire compound established so that teen pregnancies could be hidden from society. The babies that issued forth from these traumatized girls mostly disappeared into adoption agencies. I was the only black girl there, but I didn't argue with my parents' decision. It was not an unusual refuge for pregnant teenagers of the day, and it seemed like the best choice we could make at the time. I was fifteen.

The delivery was traumatic, not so much physically, but because of my fear, the intensity of birth, and my lack of knowledge about what was happening to my body. The home did not provide any pregnancy education or preparation. One minute we were doing chores or saying prayers—the next minute we were in labor and whisked off to the hospital. There was no phone available to the girls; it wasn't certain that even our parents were called. All I know is I had a very lonely labor—my parents did not make it to the hospital before the baby arrived the next day.

What a difference a doula would have made. Someone to tell me about my body's processes, what delivery would be like. Someone to squeeze my hand or make eye contact with during contractions—someone to help the doctors and nurses when the unexpected occurred. Scared does not begin to describe my feral panic. When I hear of doulas working with women to establish birthing plans and ensure that medical staff respects them, I marvel at how different pregnancies can be because of their visionary compassion.

As hard as giving birth under those lonely, terrified circumstances was, the harder moments came *after* birth, when I needed an advocate. I decided to place my son for adoption because I did not want this tortuous path to motherhood. I was in tenth grade, had college in my future, and did not want to parent my rapist's child. But everything changed when the nurses placed my son on my chest. I couldn't go through with the adoption, but I wasn't ready to parent either. I hadn't even selected a name for the child I was now going to keep.

As soon as I articulated that I wanted to raise my son,

I was assailed by the hospital, the Salvation Army home, and my parents—all of whom wanted me to stick to the plan and place my son for adoption. I had no one to listen to me. My parents eventually supported my decision. They co-parented with me through high school and college, and I recognize what a privilege it was to enjoy such strong family support.

A few years later, I made a different parenting decision under different circumstances. I had an abortion as a first-year college student. Over the years, I have witnessed women making reproductive choices under diverse life circumstances. I have escorted a few friends to abortion clinics, and I've given money to other friends who couldn't afford their procedures. To me, then, this book is a celebration of the fact that we're fortunate to live in a new era in which advocates and caregivers can center the needs of the pregnant individual regardless of the decision that person ultimately makes.

I can attest to how desperately this movement is needed. The last person I escorted to a clinic was a twelve-year-old girl still sucking her thumb who was, in all probability, the victim of childhood sexual abuse. She urgently needed a doula because her mother—likely emotionally overwhelmed herself—appeared deaf to her daughter's obvious signs of distress. A doula could have helped the mother and the daughter both—maybe even assisted them in selecting a birth control option. The mother had refused to even consider the possible future need.

Doulas provide services at the intersections of our most essential human rights: the right to give birth, the right to not give birth, and the right to safely parent children—the three cornerstones of reproductive justice. Crafted by African American women in 1994 and powerfully popularized by radical women of color, reproductive justice organizes the collective knowledge of women of color based on our pregnancy and parenting experiences. It turns that knowledge into new analyses that recognize how our own value systems based on human rights connect us to each other, and confronts the concussive impact of multiple oppressions on our reproductive lives. Racism can distort a birthing or adoption experience. Transphobia can lead to the denial of vital healthcare. Prejudice against immigrants can divide families through deportation. Misogyny can reduce pregnant women to walking wombs without rights. These are all reproductive justice issues, and doulas are the birth justice wing of our movement.

Doulas understand the unique nature of each person's situation. At the same time, they comprehend the systemic factors that affect these experiences, such as race, age, English proficiency, citizenship, gender identity, class, and the host of integrative—not additive—forces that contour pregnancy experiences. They don't shy away from naming oppressions—white supremacy, colonialism, xenophobia, homophobia, transphobia—yet they are not there to preach, but to serve. Their actions to support each and every pregnant person speak louder than any polemic on reproductive oppression or the medical industrial complex.

In a sense, these new doulas echo the full-service midwives of previous centuries. When physician-based medical care was unavailable to many people, they relied on midwives who handled births and deaths. These midwives were trusted, respected, and valued for the critical role they played in people's lives from beginning to end. Through similar compassion and dedication, contemporary doulas are creating a new tradition and demonstrating profound expressions of feminism in action. If activism is the art of making your life matter, the doulas are activists extraordinaire.

—LORETTA ROSS
Atlanta, Georgia
January 2016

Introduction
An Organization on the Fringe

In October of 2008 the Doula Project—then known as the Abortion Doula Project—held its very first volunteer training. Our mission was to educate a new generation of doulas on a burgeoning model of care: support during abortions.

As far as we knew, this was the first training of its kind; we were starting from scratch. Roughly a dozen trainees joined us that weekend. We made a motley crew: fellow reproductive justice activists, academics, close friends—all of various races, classes, sexual orientations, and gender identities.

The two of us had been attending abortions for only a few months and knew we had a lot to learn, so we invited experts in our field to lead us through workshops that covered topics like diversity awareness and physical and emotional support techniques. Halfway through our last session of the day, the trainer we'd hired, a respected abortion counselor and birth doula, made a startling announcement.

"There are lots of different ways to be doulas, I suppose," she told the assembled group. "My husband is a great parallel parking doula," she laughed gently. "But you will have to decide as a group whether or not you think it's *appropriate* to call yourselves doulas. I'm not sure it is. Just think about all the things that doulas do." She lowered her light voice slightly and tipped her chin down, very seriously. "You're not *really* doulas."

The confused trainees shifted uncomfortably in their seats as her words cut through the room. They looked to us, question marks in their eyes.

We swept in quickly, "Yes, we do all of the things that doulas do," we assured them, glancing at each other with a cringe. "Yes we are—we are doulas!"

We were stunned. We were horrified. We were pissed. We invite her into our home, and she says *this*?

The trainer left shortly after. "What the fuck was that?" someone called out.

"We are doulas; this is what we are. It's not a discussion," we repeated clumsily. Everyone nodded in agreement, unsure what to say next.

As our anger faded, it occurred to us that this trainer didn't automatically "get" what we were trying to do. Insult aside, her statement raised some important questions of mission and identity for us, ones we would be tasked with answering for years to come: What are we? Where do we belong? What do we want to become?

The Doula Project has always been an organization on the fringe. Since our inception we have struggled to figure out where exactly we "fit." Are we a healthcare organization? Political advocates? Do we all identify as feminists? Where do we place ourselves in birthing justice? How do we participate in both macro-level activism and individual direct care at once? How can we be taken seriously when we operate under a radical leadership structure and are run by unpaid volunteers? What the hell are doulas anyway?

Let's start with the easiest question. "Doula" finds its roots in the Greek word for "female slave," an unfortunate denotation that has morphed over the years into the less embattled "woman who serves." It's a word that has slowly made its way into the zeitgeist. Over time its meaning has changed and expanded to include service to women, men, transgender and gender nonconforming people, those giving birth, those having abortions, and those dying.

In the mid-twentieth century, doulas were reinvented to attend to pregnant people in the months leading up to their birth, during the birth itself, and in the days and weeks that followed the birth. They were the nonmedical caregivers in the room, the ones who would give you a massage, introduce you to a new labor position, help you take that next deep breath, offer encouragement to avoid the epidural, and listen while you emotionally processed your experience after the delivery.

In the past decade, the rise of the "abortion doula" has brought a dynamic change to the job description. These doulas took the same model of continuous, nonjudgmental support that birth doulas had become known for and moved it into the abortion clinic. In doing so, an entire population of people who had previously gone without support became recipients of a dedicated, caring presence.

Following quickly on the heels of the abortion doula came the "full-spectrum doula," a term we coined to describe a person who supports a pregnancy no matter the outcome—whether it is birth, abortion, miscarriage, or fetal anomaly. This brand of doula care typically consists of physical, emotional, educational, and spiritual support and almost always involves being present during an abortion or birth. Many full-spectrum doulas approach the work, not only from a stance of individual care and respect, but also from a deeper political conviction that anyone who becomes pregnant deserves bodily autonomy, meaningful support, and full access to quality health services. The Doula Project would come to identify as a full-spectrum organization and help define this term and its role within reproductive justice.

As legions of people around the country became interested in the work of the Doula Project, and in becoming doulas themselves, we began to ask why. What we found was a new movement in feminist activism. Young people were increasingly connecting to reproductive rights through direct service work, not just policy-advocacy methods. New pro-choice organizations and collectives were extending beyond traditional feminist advocacy groups like NARAL and NOW. Groups like Social Workers for Reproductive Justice, Nursing Students for Choice, and Medical Students for Choice, among others, were making strides to unite micro direct-care programs with macro policy initiatives.

Direct service workers have often been left on the outskirts of advocacy and social-change movements—not for lack of purpose or importance—but because they do not have a vehicle through which to channel their activism into a greater political movement. This new generation of abortion activists and service professionals was thirsty for the kind of work that could bridge the gap between local social service and broad-based social change. Full-spectrum doulas started to fill this gap; to many, the simple act of literally standing with someone during their abortion felt like a powerful political statement.

As we further investigated the sudden surge of full-spectrum doulas, we also found a group of young people longing for human connection. While much feminist and social-justice activism was taking place online, the doula movement allowed activists to connect face-to-face with people confronting the realities of what the "spectrum of choice" really means. The doula movement could be seen as a counterpoint to the online activist movement—a way to physically connect in a world that is increasingly reliant on virtual connection.

The human connection most doulas seek, however, comes with a price—being exposed to the underbelly of what pregnancy and reproductive healthcare truly look like in this country. Pregnancy, and the decision to become a parent or not, are realities that most families will confront. Yet for some people—particularly low-income people and people of color—these experiences are often silenced. Worse still, they suffer the loss of personal agency as decisions that should be private become politically and bureaucratically charged. In the current sociopolitical landscape—which features oppressive new state laws around abortion instituted by antichoice governors, high rates of cesarean sections and maternal mortality, and prohibitive healthcare costs— doulas are providing crucial support to pregnant clients and medical staff alike. Furthermore, we help give voice to the experiences of pregnant people that may otherwise go unheard.

Because of our unique hands-on relationship with healthcare institutions, full-spectrum doulas have an opportunity to challenge dominant medical and social paradigms. Ours is a quiet brand of activism: an advocacy of compassion, a watchful eye over the medical industrial complex. Most of the Doula Project doulas come to this role from the perspective of activists, both in the clients they seek to serve and in their capacity as unpaid volunteers. People frequently refer to us as "advocates." While we would not argue that point, we hope this book will show you how advocacy as a doula looks different from advocacy in other realms.

Often it simply means this: we are "holders." We hold space by creating safe, comfortable environments where our clients can be heard. We physically hold our clients through supportive and nurturing touch. We hold stories and experiences and reflect them back to our clients to help shape a memory that is meaningful. We hold abundant love for our clients and each other in times of crisis and in times of joy, even when we are little more than familiar strangers.

Telling Our Story

Our practice as doulas is a daily expression of the union between compassion and advocacy. Our story, shaped by our position as founders of the first full-spectrum doula organization and by years of experience in clinics, is both harrowing and beautiful. It is tinged with as many moments of social justice acumen as important lessons about life and love, all set within a medical framework that can feel both archaic and chaotic.

Above all, when we speak of our work, it is our stories of providing care that move and inspire people. We realize that people are drawn to personal narratives, and we recognize that these narratives are crucial to our ability to create awareness around this work and wider access to doula care. Robert Coles, author of *The Call of Stories*, writes, "Stories are renderings of life; they cannot only keep us company, but admonish us, point us in new directions, or give us the courage to stay a given course." Our stories as doulas are a window that most people don't have—stories that can give a glimpse into realities many cannot otherwise articulate, or choose to ignore, or have been too busy to notice.

Our book is a narrative about doulas and miscarriage, stillbirth, adoption, and abortion. The chapters that follow give voice to the kind of pregnancy that people don't want to talk about, the kind that is considered painful, shameful, and complicated—and, therefore, is silenced. From KCl (potassium chloride) injections in the twenty-fourth week to court-ordered C-sections in the forty-fifth hour, from tears of grief to joyful relief at the end of a first trimester abortion, it is through personal narrative that these experiences are humanized.

Though understanding systemic oppression is crucial to

the way we approach doula care, we believe that individual stories have the ability to pierce the veil covering systems that affect millions of people; they are unique but universal. We recognize that in telling the stories of our doulas, we are also telling the stories of our clients. The nature of our role means that our stories have become intertwined. As we wrote this book, we had hoped to reach each of the clients in these stories so that we could include their perspectives on the experience. When we had no way to find some of them, we struggled with including them in the book. While it's common for direct-care professionals to incorporate "case studies" into their writing and change identifying information, this practice made us uneasy.

Ultimately we consulted with trusted colleagues in the field—particularly those who have experience helping others tell their abortion stories—about how to navigate our concerns. Reproductive justice advocate and writer Renee Bracey Sherman, author of *Saying Abortion Aloud*, a guide to abortion storytelling and supporting storytellers, says:

> Sharing stories, especially abortion stories, can be an ethical gray area. Doulas want to and should be able to share their experiences of supporting people through their abortions. It's powerful to hear firsthand how to show up for someone else with compassion. However we must remember to put the needs of the patients first—we must prioritize their confidentiality, rights, and desire to share their own story on their own terms. But stories build com-

munity and alleviate isolation. That's how they serve the movement—by reminding people that they are not alone.

Storytelling, we learned, has an adhesive quality; as we share our stories, we move beyond a partnership between doulas and their clients and start to include everyone. Doulas do not approach their role in isolation. An entire lifetime has inspired us to become caregivers. When we do this work, we think about our families, our friends, the people we love. For clients, it is often the same. Melissa Madera, former full-spectrum doula and founder of *The Abortion Diary Podcast*, reminds us that the ethics and anxieties of storytelling reach clients, too—because telling a story means your narrative is documented as a kind of truth. As people describe their own experiences with abortion during Madera's interviews, they raise concerns about talking about their loved ones. They frequently ask her, "Do you think it's okay?"

When writing this book, with a few exceptions for which we received consent, we've intentionally made the dominant story and point of view that of the doula. Why is it important that we tell the stories of doulas? Because doulas are caregivers, and caregiving takes a toll. Stories from the caregiver perspective are often left out of conversations; we are supporting actors to the client's leading role. When we sign on to be caregivers, we are giving up a part of our identities for the sake of another person. Our work means that we are engaged in a deep intimacy with other people daily—the grief and joy of our clients, the doctors we work with, and each other.

As we were collecting oral histories, we realized that people rarely, if ever, have the opportunity to share their stories. The process became mutually therapeutic: we were given the privilege of listening and holding the stories for those who spoke, and in turn they often felt emotional release in letting their stories go. When we spoke with Madera about this, she articulated the symbolic gesture that happens in these exchanges, "You release the story to me, you create space for relief, and I take the story away with me, and in that way I become a part of the story, too."

So much of doula work is that transference of story and the transference of emotional burden that goes with it. Physician David Grimes has written at length about the emotional transference exchanged between patient and provider during abortion. According to Grimes, in the act of providing the abortion, the provider accepts and takes away the patient's emotional burden. This book represents a narrative version of that exchange—doing doula work all day, every day, means that we become filled with stories. At the end of the day, we do not just bear witness to someone else's story, we become a part of that story and that story becomes a part of us. We try to receive emotional burden for as long as we can, but the relief of that burden comes with our own sharing. It's cyclical. We found that writing this book became more than a process to document our stories—it was accidentally therapeutic. Ultimately, writing and listening to these stories and to one another gave us a new space to give and receive compassionate care.

How to Read This Book

Our hope is to bring readers into the world of care where we exist. We want to engage you with the narratives of our beginnings, our moments of greatest success, and the places where we've learned our most valuable lessons. To do this, we have woven together our own narratives as the Doula Project founders with those of other doulas, former clients, medical providers, and allies.

In order to gather the stories of those who have helped shape the organization, we conducted dozens of interviews. Many were done in the tradition of "oral histories." A few of these oral histories would become the basis for entire chapters in the book. For these histories, we spent time gathering intimate details and engaging the storytellers in sensory exercises to craft a rich and accurate narrative. We then read the text aloud with them, inviting them into the editing process. We have used first-person narrative, third-person narrative, and direct quotations to write this book—following the style of creative nonfiction, a genre that merges literary elements with factual, biographical information.

We have changed the names of some of our clients, allies, and partner organizations, as well as certain locations where stories take place. We've also changed the names of most of our clinic sites to protect the availability of their services. (When it comes to abortion care, fame rarely brings anything good.)

We believe you will get the most out of the book by reading it in order from front to back. Descriptions of medical procedures and interventions, laws and policies, and introductions to recurring doulas are sequenced in this manner. Should you need this book as a reference guide, however, we have also created multiple sections with different topics so that you can easily flip to what interests you most—doulas supporting other doulas, birth stories, or direct-care activism, for example. In every section, multiple themes are covered, ranging from adoption politics to ambivalent feelings about abortion to provider burnout and more.

This book is the creative memoir of an organization—a story of what it means to be a doula, a story about giving love and getting it back through this rare, uniquely beautiful exchange. At its core, it's a story about humans trying to take care of each other in a world where that often gets lost. Those who have ever cared for anyone will relate.

Part I
The Beginning

A Great Idea

The Abortion Doula Project was a great idea.

It was one of those brilliant shining stars that catches your eye from high above, the kind you want to reach up and grab with both hands, make a wish on. And this was it in all its profound simplicity: people having abortions should have continuous and nonjudgmental physical, emotional, and educational support just like people giving birth. For one year, between the summers of 2007 and 2008, we floated on our big, beautiful idea, lifting it up bright and glowing into a cloudless sky.

The idea was conceived at the NYC Birth Coalition meeting, a local attempt to bring abortion and birth activists together in one room—something that didn't normally happen. That day, Lauren Mitchell, Mary Mahoney, and Miriam Zoila Pérez, the Doula Project's founders, all stood up and said, "We want to be *abortion doulas.*"

Words of encouragement fluttered through the air, the group nodded and smiled at each other as the idea dawned.

Maybe this will be the next "big thing," their reactions seemed to say.

The three of us circled each other curiously. We had met briefly before at some point or another—the New York repro scene was relatively small. We decided to grab lunch after the meeting. We walked to Zuccotti Park to eat our deli fare and jumped into how we might start an abortion doula program here in the city.

We had each entered the reproductive justice fold in the early to mid-2000s and were trained under its holistic justice-based framework created by women of color in the 1990s, with Loretta Ross spearheading the conversation. Often, the feminist movement of the 1960s is associated with a reproductive rights framework—the right to choose when, how, and with whom someone has children. Reproductive justice takes that movement further, bringing together intersections of identity to form a definition of social justice hinged on lived experiences—especially lived experiences of women of color. It analyzes and exposes the intersections—including gender, race, sexual orientation, and access to resources—that affect how a person makes decisions and whether that person has meaningful choices around reproductive health. Reproductive justice looks not only at the right one has to an abortion but also one's right to have a child and to parent that child.

Connecting the right to give birth and parent to the right to an abortion was a groundbreaking concept that would greatly influence the mission of the Doula Project (which would become our official name within a year).

Full-spectrum care, the cornerstone of our organization, was a direct descendant of the reproductive justice framework and bolstered the stance that abortion should not stand alone, that it is one part of a person's entire reproductive life. The same individual may have an abortion, give birth, and then have a miscarriage. The point we feminists wanted to make was no longer only, "I'm having an abortion." It was now, "I am pregnant. This is what I *choose* to do for this pregnancy. This is what I am *able* to do. Next time, I might choose something different. Can I get some care and support for *this* pregnancy's path?"

Full-spectrum care acknowledged the experience of being pregnant—whether for four weeks or nine months—not just the outcome of the pregnancy. Somehow this idea seemed new. Aimée Thorne-Thomsen, former executive director of the Pro-Choice Public Education Project (PEP), early advisor to the Doula Project, and current vice president for Strategic Partnerships at Advocates for Youth, remembers:

> It felt like there were more conversations about the end result of pregnancy. We would talk a lot about abortion or birth control, we would talk about things *around* pregnancy, but not pregnancy itself. And at the point you all were going to launch, it was like, huh, there's a process here that we skip over in the field all the time: the actual pregnancy.

We were compelled to do this work because we wanted to see and feel the changes we were trying to create. The reproductive justice movement was home to us, and we were well aware of the debt we owed to the intellectual and political framework it created, which opened the door for us to dive into this project. We were standing on the shoulders of giants, women in the field who were changing both policy and the messages being presented in media. As a result they changed the lives of countless people, who started receiving better care and more acknowledgment of the state of their care.

We also looked back to the 1960s and early 1970s, the time before *Roe v. Wade* was decided, when women still had to obtain abortions illegally in most states. We discovered Jane, the underground abortion network in Chicago that helped more than eleven thousand women receive safe abortions between 1969 and 1973. Jane was known for its radical feminist politics and DIY spirit. Members of Jane put together pop-up abortion clinics in whatever nice apartments they could find, they did extensive counseling and phone support, they provided post-abortion care—and often were the abortion providers. What we were most struck by, though, was how much support and care was exchanged between the members of Jane and their clients who had little to no anesthesia to offset the pain. Thinking about how this support played out, Laura Kaplan, author of *The Story of Jane* and one of the coordinators of the Jane Collective, reflects, "How you behave toward another person and what you do for her affects her view of herself."

Kaplan describes the Jane Collective as mixing abundant idealism and social responsibility. They were responding to a pressing need in the community, saying, "We saw all of these problems, and we felt like abortion access was something we could actually do something about." They learned quickly what we would also learn quickly: that direct care means you do not put good against perfect. "We were very focused on the here and now," she says. People would call needing abortions and needing them fast. Most of the time, they weren't able to pay much, if anything at all, so Jane worked through the energy of volunteers, with a handful of paid staff who were doing the heavy lifting of coordination and procedures. An elaborate yet flexible process was set up to ensure that Jane would be able to operate efficiently and under the radar of the law. But doing this work on the fringes of legal and medical systems highlighted that no amount of planning and theorizing would be able to anticipate the messy reality of working with people during abortions.

We set out to translate the reproductive justice framework into a more direct-care-oriented approach, using pieces of what Jane did as a model. The reproductive justice movement promotes the idea that, in a lifetime, a person might experience the full spectrum of reproductive health decisions, that these decisions are linked to other intersecting factors in their life, and that any decision made should be respected and protected. So what did this actually look like on the ground for pregnant people? How was this lived out during their pregnancies?

Cofounder Miriam Zoila Pérez (who goes by Pérez), founded the blog *Radical Doula* and wrote *The Radical Doula Guide: A Political Primer for Full-Spectrum Pregnancy and Birth Support*. Pérez reflects:

Starting a program to support people during abortions just made so much sense to me. Of course doulas can and should use their skills during a different pregnancy outcome. Why wouldn't we? I also appreciated the potential political impacts of even the phrase "abortion doula." I knew that it would push at the silos between abortion and birth, and hopefully push the birth activist world to talk about abortion and miscarriage.

As we laid down the bones of our mission, a simple but strong skeleton formed, built largely on our own personal value systems and what we had uncovered fighting for reproductive equality over the years. We quickly agreed that the clients we most wanted to serve were the ones who may not have easy access to social support during pregnancy or who could not afford to go to the private clinics or fancy hospitals with the most resources. Because New York is a very culturally diverse city with enormous disparities in wealth and class status often based on the color of a person's skin, primary language, or age, we knew we would primarily be serving women of color, immigrants, and young people.

We wanted our service to be free to all people who needed it, something we would become known for throughout the doula world. Doulas are often reserved for a more affluent crowd—their service isn't cheap and is not typically covered by health insurance. We believed all pregnant people deserved this kind of support regardless of their financial status. In order to do this with little to no funding of our own, we, like the Jane Collective before us, decided we would create a volunteer network. Lauren and Pérez had already attended numerous volunteer births as doulas, and Mary had been an AmeriCorps VISTA. We all felt passionate about the power of volunteerism, of the emotional intimacy that arises from our work when it's based on a fiery commitment to the cause rather than on compensation.

As the years went on, however, we would learn that in New York City "volunteerism" often equated itself to "middle class" and even more often to "white middle class." Abortions typically took place during the day, during the week, when many people could not afford to miss work. Though we were and continue to be in awe of the incredible caring capacity of the doulas who joined, we cringed at the thought of creating another racialized, class-based hierarchy in medicine. We would struggle to diversify our base in the face of a meager budget and ever-growing client and clinic needs. (As this book is being written, we have passed our first budget to pay abortion doulas a small stipend.)

As we were coming together in 2007, the birth doula community in New York City was at the cusp of an explosion of a new generation of doulas. In addition to the ongoing abortion debate, the heat of the "home vs. hospital" birth argument was at its zenith. Maternal mortality and C-section rates were on the rise and people were speaking up. Abby Epstein's eye-opening documentary *The Business of Being Born* was released soon after we became birth doulas. Suddenly, it seemed that everyone had a "birth plan" and everything was "natural"—natural products, natural labors, and natural approaches to parenting.

Meanwhile, a few months prior to the NYC Birth Coalition meeting, National Advocates for Pregnant Women (NAPW) convened a conference that brought birth and abortion activists together in one room for the first time in most of our memories. The NAPW's 2007 National Summit to Ensure Health and Humanity of Pregnant and Birthing Women offered a crucial platform for activists and was in some ways iconoclastic: it engaged with reproductive justice activists as well as with staunchly anti-abortion birth activists. It was trying to build alliances across political dominions in a way we hadn't seen before—for example, it created contact between abortion providers and birth activists who feared that they would go to hell for sharing space with them. But as Lynn Paltrow, founder and executive director of NAPW, discussed at length with both communities, the "justification for locking women up and forcing them to have court-ordered C-sections stems from the same legal justifications developed for restricting abortions. [In other words] there is no difference in the legal theories used to restrict abortion and those used to justify forcing a woman to have cesarean surgery."

In trying to connect both communities, Lynn describes the work of the NAPW conference as "pragmatic" because both communities were advocating for the same women—just at different points in their reproductive lives. She also hoped that bringing the two activist communities together would "detoxify the abortion debate by making it richer and more complex [and] by saying, you can't just talk about ending a pregnancy."

According to activist and scholar Marlene Gerber Fried,

director of the Civil Liberties and Public Policy program (CLPP) at Hampshire College, "Historically, the frame of choice wasn't about having children, but rather the choice not to. And while there was much overlap in individual players and organizations who worked between the two worlds, for decades they were usually very siloed."

CLPP was also instrumental in bringing together voices from both movements at their annual conference. The CLPP Conference facilitates one of the largest platforms for activists, especially young activists, in the country, often influencing themes and ideas among organizers for the year to come. In 2007 a number of doulas were invited to speak at CLPP. Those talks followed the conference's Abortion Speak-Out, a night where people share stories about their own abortions. The Speak-Out is known for being a beautiful space for those who come to listen and those who come to share. The Speak-Out would be a huge inspiration to us, in many ways a cornerstone of our compassionate practice, as we developed as an organization.

Between the burgeoning success of *The Business of Being Born*, the connection reproductive justice advocates were facilitating between birth and abortion, and a new activist-flavored onslaught of birth doulas saturating New York City, the timing for the Abortion Doula Project seemed perfect. We continued to formulate our mission.

Pérez says now:

In that first year of creating [the Doula Project], I remember a lot of exploring what it would look like to take the skills and role of a birth doula and apply it to the abortion context. I remember a lot of hypothesizing about what someone having an abortion would want from a doula. We were wrong about a lot of the assumptions we made, but it makes sense that we were wrong. We were really charting new territory.

With this new territory came several months of starts and stops. We were all young, busting our asses at our full-time jobs, navigating a city that left us worn to the bone at each day's end. Weeks would pass, and the Abortion Doula Project would feel like nothing but a misty memory. One day, Pérez announced she was moving to Washington, DC, to pursue new personal and professional opportunities. Unsure of whether to proceed without her, the two of us (Lauren and Mary) met up to determine the fate of the organization. We decided that we were finally "gonna do this," although we would now approach it as a duo.

To us, and to many others, the idea of providing compassionate emotional, physical, informational support was intuitive, whether we called it "doula care" or any other name. We knew that there were social workers, counselors, nurses, doctors, clinic escorts, and many others who were providing this care before "abortion doulas" became an official concept. In fact, there are some clinics like Preterm in Cleveland, Ohio, and Choices in Memphis, Tennessee, that hired patient support people as soon as they opened. But we also knew that at many clinics, offering adequate support at the time of an abortion could be a matter of luck and timing—whoever happens to be working that day, and whoever happens to have time.

So we figured the best way to support clinics and reach the most clients would be to partner with a clinic itself. Typically, in a traditional relationship between birth doula and client, a doula would meet a client outside the confines of a hospital and accompany her into the labor and delivery room without any official volunteer or staff status within that hospital. Abortion clinics, however, usually prohibit friends or family from joining clients in their exam rooms for procedures to ensure the safety of clients and staff alike. Moreover, we did not expect that an individual seeking a pregnancy termination would ask for this type of support given the stigma attached to abortion and the limited time period involved. Not to mention, people were barely even familiar with doulas for birth, let alone this totally new concept—how would they even know to ask?

We went in search of a clinic to pilot our project. We weren't exactly sure where to start. We cold-called a few local facilities, sent some letters. No response. We spoke to midwives and obstetricians who tepidly expressed support but didn't offer abortion services at their practices. We went back to what we knew—the reproductive justice movement. We traveled the country, speaking about abortion doulas at meetings and conferences, often connecting with Pérez along the way. As the months rolled on, it seemed that the Abortion Doula Project was destined to remain only "a great idea."

Though not totally defeated, we were officially frustrated.

We knew feminist leaders, young and old. We had all the right connections in our field. Why were we turned away? Why couldn't we find anyone to partner with? Why couldn't we connect with the people inside the clinic walls?

This is when we first started to see the disconnect that often exists between the advocacy and direct-care worlds. Sure, we knew the executive director of Advocates for Youth in Washington, DC. That didn't mean we knew the local abortion provider practicing in our neighborhood clinic in New York City. On top of that, we realized that even though politically "birthing justice" was under the umbrella of "reproductive justice," birth and abortion were often clinically separated from one another.

Fortunately for us, there were a handful of other activists and national groups walking the line between advocacy and direct care. We discovered groups that, for years, had been promoting a message of care similar to ours. We began to connect with them.

Aspen Baker was a big supporter of ours from the start. As founder and executive director of Exhale, a postabortion hotline that promoted a "pro-voice" framework, Baker had spent years listening to the stories of people who had abortions and bringing those stories into the public sphere. In the summer of 2008, she asked Mary to speak about the abortion doula philosophy of care at a pro-voice event at the Guttmacher Institute in Manhattan. When Exhale was being developed, the founders had briefly considered training doulas before deciding on a talk-line. Baker remembers "feeling really excited and really proud and really supportive of the idea [of abortion doulas] and glad that someone else was going to make something real and tangible and needed for women."

During her presentation, Mary announced that the Abortion Doula Project was looking for a clinic to partner with, as she often did when she spoke in public. Normally, nothing came of the announcement other than some much-appreciated words of encouragement. But at the end of the meeting that day, two young women approached Mary. Their names were Dahlia and Sarah, and they were the interns of Dr. B. Dahlia came from CLPP's intern program, and, together, she and Sarah were invested in finding creative approaches to improving reproductive health outcomes for women. They thought Dr. B might want to meet the founders of the Abortion Doula Project. She was the director of the Reproductive Choices clinic at City Hospital, and this was exactly the project she had been looking for.

City Hospital ran a small abortion service that focused on complicated cases, either medically or financially speaking. Pregnant people were referred there if they had a high-risk pregnancy that a freestanding clinic could not manage or if they were unable to pay full price for their abortions or qualify for Medicaid. At the point when we were introduced to the clinic they were expanding their service and looking for greater support systems for their clients.

The clinical coordinators, who served as the primary abortion counselors, were typically responsible for attending procedures with clients at City Hospital; Dr. B wanted to make sure someone was always there. But as their workload increased, the clinic realized they needed someone else to fill that gap. Dr. B remembers, "Before [the doulas] it was fine, but [the counselors] were just really busy because there's such a high demand for services. [The doulas] took a huge burden off of them."

The day we entered City Hospital for our first meeting, we were beyond nervous. Mary had a terrible headache. Lauren, who had woken up at three in the morning for no good reason, mulled over her second cup of coffee and prayed she wouldn't pass out at random. We were both wearing khakis and button-downs for probably the first time in our lives. We looked like 1990s Gap clerks. It was our first big chance to be abortion doulas: we couldn't blow it.

Little did we know, Dr. B had already green-lighted the project on the recommendation of Dahlia and Sarah. As long as Melissa, the clinic coordinator agreed, we were in. This would be our first lesson in the power the abortion counselor has in the clinic, the way in which they hold the service together.

We met Melissa, Sarah, and Dahlia in an exam room, one that would become the site of hundreds of meetings with our clients. Both parties tittered with excitement, the energy crackled, electric. It was like the beginning of a great first date. We all knew immediately we had found "the one."

Within ten minutes Melissa was handing us the clinic schedule for the following week. We blinked. After a year of trying, our work finally began.

Dr. B says today that the clinic was "really the ideal situation" for introducing doulas. She reflects:

Dr. M, the previous clinic director, had started a clinic [through the hospital] that was kind of a freestanding unit, and we didn't have anesthesia. So we just had ourselves, who were trained to offer conscious sedation, but nobody was completely asleep. The nurse was also super busy getting all the details medically done so having an extra support person for the patient was just really phenomenal. It made things better for all of us. You were so incredibly dedicated. There were [patients] who were coming from far away, some with absolutely no support people, so having that support was amazing.

Those early years of existence would test us beyond what we could imagine, in the most wonderful ways as well as the most challenging. "I remember how excited and nervous you all were," Thorne-Thomsen says today. "You already realized you were gonna hit some bumps. You were breaking orthodoxies, and I think you knew that. And so there was an excitement, but also, like, 'How are people gonna receive this? How is this gonna go down?'"

Pushback

In a 2010 *Slate* article entitled "What's An Abortion Doula?" writer Marisa Meltzer opined that abortion doulas "seemed unnecessary" and that they "don't do anything during an abortion that a friend or clinic worker couldn't do." The piece went on to question whether women were "so fragile that they need to hire a complete stranger to hold their hand at the doctor's."

When we created the Abortion Doula Project, we

understood that the "abortion doula" was a provocative idea. We knew that we would face pushback, that the world might not "get it" right away. "Any new or different idea takes some time to get used to," we comforted ourselves.

There were those who didn't see the distinction between us and a clinic escort or recovery volunteer, between a counselor or someone who "just stands there and holds a hand." There were the more traditional pro-choice groups and activists who would express concern about our acknowledgment of the emotion that accompanies an abortion. We had been fed narratives through our activist work that many people felt "empowered" by their abortions. But our very presence in the procedure room undermined that message by hinting that abortion might be physically painful or people might have complicated feelings about it. Mostly what we saw from people having abortions was a nuanced mix of mourning and relief. We would rarely hear that our clients regretted their procedures, nor would we hear them speak of it in empowering terms. But when we talked about all of this, it often wasn't received by the pro-choice community the way we expected it to be.

Supporting a client before, during, and after an abortion, being a nonjudgmental presence and having no agenda other than that, was a departure from the standard pro-choice framework. We were coming from advocacy and policy backgrounds, connected to the people creating the abortion rights messages in the United States. We knew that acknowledging complicated feelings about abortion was going to be a delicate task and that being real about what an abortion actually *looked* like would be even more delicate. Asserting that someone might *need* support during an abortion? Forget it. Those were acknowledgments that many felt could be dangerous to the policies and laws in place that protect our right to choose.

Frequently, there was concern that we could be feeding the antichoice movement with our perspectives. Baker reflects on this sentiment, "Before Exhale started, the most prominent people who were talking about post-abortion feelings were pro-life." There had been a few pro-choice projects here and there that had considered this perspective—such as the books *Peace after Abortion* (1996) and *The Healing Choice* (1997), the November Gang, and Anne Baker's work at the Hope Clinic in St. Louis—but these were "few and far between and did not have wide pro-choice support."

The common pro-choice refrain was "most women feel relief"—and nothing else—and pro-choice advocates rejected the idea of a "postabortion syndrome" (characterized by stress, anxiety, and depression) that had been coined by pro-life organizations. It was assumed that anyone who talked about abortion feelings, especially difficult ones like sadness or grief, had been bamboozled by pro-life extremists. In truth, a political strategy *had* been developed to make abortion an unthinkable option for women. Part of making it unthinkable was to say that it was something women might regret, and to save women from the pain of regret, they should not have the choice.

Today, we have organizations like the I Had an Abortion Project, the Abortion Conversation Project, and Sea Change. We have films like *I Had an Abortion* and *Silent Choices*. We have innovations such as the 1 in 3 Campaign, *The*

Abortion Diary Podcast, and Angie Jackson live-tweeting her procedure. We have abortion speak-outs happening all over the country. Because of this, it may seem obvious that acknowledging the complexities of abortion is the direction the movement should head in—in fact, it is already headed there. Ten years ago, creating direct service work within this nuance was more complicated. Thorne-Thomsen reflects, "In some ways, the movement either moves glacially or at the speed of light, sometimes both, so it feels like nothing's changing, nothing's changing, and then overnight everything has changed at once. And I think storytelling, narrative, and putting out a broader idea of what an abortion experience is looks dramatically different since the Doula Project started."

Each time an article diminishing us was published, we were surprised. Wouldn't acknowledging the human element in abortion reduce the stigma of the procedure? Wasn't our mutual goal to make it less shameful and secretive? Wouldn't sharing the individual reality of abortion serve to uphold the value and safety of the procedure? How could there be such disconnect between real people's lived experiences and the pro-choice messages coming from the media and major pro-choice organizations?

But the disconnect between direct care and policy advocacy was real. As we were conceptualizing the Doula Project we experienced this ourselves. We went into the clinic with our own baggage from the advocacy world, our own assumptions. For one, we assumed all of our clients would identify with the word "abortion." We quickly met people having miscarriages and those who felt unsafe using that word, so we starting saying "procedure" instead, or reflecting whatever language our clients used. We also met clients who didn't identify as women, and so we became more intentional about using the term "pregnant people." Additionally, we had assumed we would be engaging in tons of postabortion care—as it turned out that need was never expressed by our clients. Pérez reflects, "I think advocates often make the mistake of assuming they know what the people they are trying to advocate for need. Direct care offers an opportunity to put those assumptions aside and actually listen to the needs of the person."

While understanding the important macro connections and implications of direct care, its primary goal was individual support. The policy world didn't necessarily want to silence abortion stories, but they were selective about the ones that should be shared: their primary goal was to protect the legal right to an abortion. For example, we were much more likely to hear a story of late-term abortion that focused on the health of the mother or the baby than we were to hear about a woman who didn't know whether she wanted an abortion until later in her term or found out she was pregnant during her twentieth week. We were also more likely to hear a story of a woman who felt empowered by her abortion than one who felt ambivalent or regretful about it.

We would learn that the two factions of the work would sometimes rub against each other. People have emotions about their abortions, and they aren't always what political movements want to hear. To this end, Baker notes that we should focus on caring about women, not just about abortion:

When someone truly cares about women they are open to hearing what women want to say about their own abortions (whether they are pro-choice or pro-life or neither), but when the care is primarily about securing or ending the legal right to abortion then there is great concern about what women say about their own abortions. If we stick with caring about women and we commit to doing it fiercely and publicly, with respect for their unique differences, faults and imperfections, then we don't have to make choices about the political relevancy of their story or their feelings. We don't have to edit and rework. We can just accept.

Many beyond the abortion rights movement were not prepared for the paradigm shift that was happening, particularly our closest critics: medical staff. They were about to let another person into the room, and to what end? Who were these abortion doulas anyway? Nurses and counselors held pieces of the doula role, with other tasks that usually took priority, and from the start we had to distinguish our role from theirs and make sure we did not take the joy of client care away from them. We learned much of how to become abortion doulas by observing nurses and counselors in action. We shared intimate space with them and witnessed the same procedures, the same client responses. We ultimately would form a community of care with them in which we all supported each other through our primary tasks.

The pro-choice and medical communities were kind in comparison to the birth community. We thought everyone was "progressive" like us—by which we meant quite simply "pro-choice." We were wrong. Many in the birth community were affronted not only by the abortion work we were doing but by the very idea that we would expand the doula name in this way. There were those who were skeptical—"You're not *really* doulas," as that birth and abortion activist famously told us at our first training—and those who outright opposed us, mostly the pro-life birth community contingent.

Lauren, Pérez, and Aimee Thorne-Thomsen had been to the NAPW conference in Atlanta that winter and had seen this tension firsthand. Thorne-Thomsen remembers, "You were either an abortion rights activist or a birth activist, and we are not the same; we are not community. Even as an abortion activist I remember feeling completely alienated from the birth rights people, and I couldn't believe this chasm exists, but it does." As a full-spectrum doula organization, we would find ourselves managing either side of this equation throughout our existence.

Today

So much of how we started was about being in the right place at the right time. Once we got the go-ahead to be in our first clinic, we spent a lot of energy sprinting from one end of the hospital to the other. We followed doctors through crowds, trying to figure out where and when we would meet our clients on any given day. We had to stick to our clients like glue, or else they would be called into a procedure and the clinic staff would forget that a doula was wandering the halls, looking for her client. We knew we had turned a corner the day we got an annoyed phone call from a clinic nurse who said, "We can't start the procedure because the doula is running late. Where is she?"

Having a doula present during an abortion is no longer "icing on the cake"—our clinics consider us an important part of their infrastructure. There is now an institutional acknowledgement that having a doula is part of a standard of care for many pregnant people, which is underscored by the fact that the doulas have been present in our clinics since before many of the doctors we work with were hired. Residents and medical students are regularly trained to do procedures with a doula in the room.

Nearly a decade later, we have served tens of thousands of clients and trained close to a thousand abortion doulas around the country. Today, it's hard to find anyone on the pro-choice spectrum opposed to abortion doulas. Baker says:

The Doula Project is unique in that it has a record of real success. You have done more than just talk about change, you have created real change in women's lives and in the lives of people who work at clinics. It's amazing that it has been done by volunteers, and that alone is something tremendous to offer the world as a message. It is absolutely the kind of culture that we can and should create.

Pérez expands on this:

I think there has been a tectonic shift in both [birth and abortion] movements, which full-spectrum doulas definitely get some credit for. Both movements are talking about birth and abortion in ways they weren't before. Both movements are being pushed to see the full spectrum of our reproductive lives. I see [full-spectrum] doulas as an incredible bridge, and I think we've been able to practice direct care while also [pushing] advocacy movements to broaden their lens.

On a national level, we have supported dozens of groups interested in doing full-spectrum doula work, and trained hundreds of activists. The "rise of the doula" is present in reproductive justice everywhere. Marlene Gerber Fried, who teaches at Hampshire College in addition to her work at the Civil Liberties and Public Policy program, remarks that she is "really struck by the heightened interest of younger advocates in doula work. Even among the cohort of students I've been working with, *many* want to be doulas. They're coming into a class about abortion but they all want to be doing birth work. This is new. And it has a lot to do with the advocacy in the birth justice movement such as the Doula Project. It's made a huge difference in drawing new energy to that work."

Fried continues, "The spectrum idea is just perfect because it forces the erasure of the bright line that divides the women who have abortions and the women who have babies. Anything that can undermine that misconception is important to the reproductive justice movement." Direct service work can provide young activists with plenty of gratification, as well. "Policy change is such a long road to walk," Fried acknowledges. "At the end of the day, seeing something through like a birth allows a young idealist to hang in there for the work that is the longer haul, and that's what I think is really great."

Those first years, we took missteps. We tripped and fell down, bruised our knees, scratched our elbows. We got back up. We learned how to frame our work in ways that were responsible to our clients, clinics, and the world of policy advocacy. We learned to appreciate that we would not be the first or last people to do this work. We created a purposeful position and named it, giving people something to hold on to. But mostly, we kept our heads down and served our clients. That's what this work is all about.

Look But Don't Touch
Mary and Maria

"You can start now." Dr. B smiles over at me expectantly as Ann snaps latex gloves on her hands and pulls them to her elbows. I move closer to the procedure table and touch its cool blue vinyl with the tips of my fingers, my other hand clenched tightly at my side. Maria's eyes flutter open as she feels my presence.

"*¿Cómo estás?*" I whisper, folding my five-ten frame to be near my client.

"*Bien*," she mouths back, then stares at the ceiling.

I follow her gaze and take in the room, a large rectangle, clean and open and somehow beautiful to me. At my back the entrance is concealed by a patterned curtain that circles around door, adding a layer of privacy for the client. Next to the door is a sink, the kind with foot pedals. The walls are lined with windowed cabinets, filled with the medications and medical supplies needed for a D and C, including chucks, gauze, gloves, sanitizer, antiseptic, and dozens of wrapped flexible curettes of various sizes.

The procedure table, where Maria lies, sits toward the back of the room. A white paper barrier rests between her and the slick vinyl. Her legs remain flat across the table, not yet fitted into the metal stirrups dangling at its sides. Tucked into the basket that holds the blood pressure cuff behind Maria is a box of tissues, a staple of doula care. At the foot of the table is a tray wrapped in soft, sterile cloth. I would come to know its contents well, their curves and sheen a second nature to me: dilators, clamps, sharp curettes, forceps, speculums, and long needles to reach into the cervix.

My attention rests on Ann, the head nurse, who is standing opposite me. Ann appears disinterested in me. She avoids eye contact as if she can sense I am seeking her approval, that I need something from her. I desperately want her to like me in a way that makes me feel twelve years old again, meeting my sixth grade teacher for the first time. This dynamic is established within seconds of my arrival, and in a way, Ann does become one of my teachers.

As I hover awkwardly near Maria, I realize I know very little about her. This unsettles me. I imagine the next fifteen minutes to be intimate, overwhelming. We are bound together by a few square feet; our bodies nearly touch, we breathe the same air. We had met briefly during precounseling earlier in the week, yet my mind at this point is a sea of facts and faces, times and names. My own ego swims and splashes through them all until my eyes are squinted and blurred, and I can only see myself pooled at the center.

Pop music plays softly on the portable radio, and Dr. B's metal instruments clink on the procedure tray as Maria breathes deeply at my side. This combination of sounds would become a part of my being as a doula. Warm morning sun pours through a picture window and down onto my client and me. The blinds are raised, revealing a fifteen-story drop, and I watch the cars multiply on the highway outside, stuck in the Manhattan commute. The river flows just beyond, and I try to make out the silhouette of my own apartment building on the other side in Brooklyn. I picture myself tonight on my roof under the sticky August moon looking back at City Hospital.

I stand above Maria, unsure of my next move. To say that my mind went blank would imply that I had some sort of plan that I had momentarily forgotten. But there isn't a plan, not really. Only a purpose: to help this woman feel safe and supported during her abortion. Whether or not I know how to do that, I am about to find out.

"I'm a doula."
   "A what?"
   "A *doo*-lah."
   "Huh?"
   "D-o-u-l-a. I attend births and abortions."
   "Oh! Wow! That's amazing!"
So have begun many conversations in the lives of full-spectrum doulas. While doulas are all Lauren and I have thought about for the better part of the last decade, we are never surprised when we meet someone who has never heard of them. Even in 2016, many small towns and big cities still have no knowledge of or access to doulas. We attribute this

in part to the abysmal state of reproductive healthcare in our country, the dearth of resources available for women to have an empowered and woman-centered pregnancy experience. More than that, we believe it is reflective of how society feels about women, about what they deserve and don't deserve—especially when pregnant.

Pregnant people are not to be trusted. This message is deeply ingrained in our culture. It's everywhere: in our laws, in our media outlets, in our homes. It's rooted in the patriarchal fear of female power and sexuality, and its pervasiveness reaches into the psyches of women themselves.

I can relate. Coming of age in white, working-class southern Indiana, a swath of the country where conservative roots grow into all its children—long before the Religious Freedom Restoration Act and Purvi Patel*—I was terrified of anything having to do with sex or my body. With good reason I thought: *I could get pregnant.* And that would be the worst thing that ever happened to me; pregnant girls dropped out of school and stayed in Smalltown, Indiana.

In the spring of 1995 I sat in my seventh grade health class, attention rapt as two high school seniors, a girl and a boy, gave me my first lesson in sex. She played varsity volleyball and had dated my friend's older brother. Her skin glowed gold as though she had just emerged from a tanning

---

* Religious Freedom Restoration Act: an Indiana Senate bill signed into law in 2015 that, in a nutshell, asserts that individuals and companies may use their religion as a defense in denying services to others. The LGBTQ community has been particularly targeted by this law. Purvi Patel: a pregnant woman who was charged with feticide and child neglect and sentenced to twenty years in prison for allegedly inducing her own miscarriage.

bed, and thin blond streaks ran through dark, gelled hair. Her raspy voice was confident and a little bored, as if she'd had this conversation a million times before. "Sex," she began with authority. He wore a letterman's jacket and didn't say much.

My best friend Meredith sat next to me, passing notes and rolling her eyes. Meredith already knew about sex, at least theoretically. She'd had boyfriends for years. She was "wanted." I was completely virginal and had only gotten my period that summer. At its inauguration Meredith had been over, and we sat on the edge of my claw-foot tub in the upstairs bathroom—door locked—while she told me about tampons. I was horrified at the thought of sticking something in my vagina. I went to find my mom. She gave me a big hug and an even bigger pad. Meredith took me for a walk to try to ease the cramps, the giant pad making a deafening noise with each step. We passed by the houses of boys we had crushes on. She was always appalled by my choices in love: "Mary! No!" Even with my latest crimson leap into "womanhood" we both knew they would never be more than a fantasy: I was not having sex.

There was a singular view of premarital sex in my hometown: *Don't do it.* That's what the high school seniors were preaching on this sunny day in southern Indiana: "You are worth waiting for!" They gave me a sticker to prove it. I eagerly stuck it to the cover of my notebook.

This message of abstinence hovered over my Christian community, a town that became quiet as a ghost on Sunday mornings. I myself went to worship the Lord every now and then. My mom even taught Sunday school to the pre-K crowd at a stuffy church attended by the hundred or so rich people in our town—but mostly she did it to throw an extra twenty-five bucks a week in our family coffer. In church, God was the one whispering, "*No premarital sex.*" I don't remember ever thinking much about God. If anything, I wasn't a fan because he reminded me of the way the snooty old ladies in pews looked down on me, my brother, and my sister. I had no idea at the time that a big part of my adulthood would be dedicated to navigating God and spirituality as a doula.

As the years passed, I learned I was far from a "good girl." I had run drunkenly from the cops through my fair share of cornfields, smoked cigarettes on the floor of my car during lunch period. But God or no God, sex still scared me. Sexually transmitted diseases? Pregnancy? Getting stuck in Indiana? I chose to keep my legs tightly closed.

By the time I was a high school junior, it was 1998 and the welfare reform law had set in motion an abstinence-only campaign valued at $50 million per year. In other words, still no premarital sex—no how, no way. I became a "Lifesaver," along with many of my friends. We went from class to class and school to school, showing photos of genital herpes and pregnant teenagers to underclassman. "Do *NOT* have sex!" we told them gravely. The words *abortion, birth control,* and even *birth* were never uttered. (Not long into the program, rumors started flying that several of the Lifesavers were giving blow jobs, among other activities. It became difficult for anyone to take us seriously.)

My parents ignored the Lifesavers aspect of my school

life. If anything they were confused. They were former hippies, rare liberal birds from "up North." "You're a *feminist!*" my dad would tell me. I didn't experience his claim as a compliment. I was convinced my dad just thought I was too opinionated or weird or bitchy. I had no concept of feminism at that point. It just wasn't part of the vocabulary of my youth.

Meanwhile, Meredith and I drifted apart. She got a serious boyfriend, and I began socializing with the "party" crowd. The night of high school graduation we got together to go to one last party. Despite my loathing for my hometown, money was tight, and I was planning to stick around for a few more years, live with my dad, work my minimum wage job as a Subway "sandwich artist," and attend community college. Meredith was off to Purdue. She couldn't wait to get out of there. "I fucking hate this place!" she yelled. Our car was a whizzing dot on the high school's security cameras. I was sitting next to her smoking, silently sticking my middle finger out the passenger window.

We didn't see each other again that summer. I got a call from her halfway through spring semester of our freshman year: "I'm pregnant. I'm coming back home." We spent the next six months watching *Felicity*, eating ice cream, and being best friends again. Meredith was having the baby, unlike another friend of ours, Shannon, who was also pregnant.

I met with Shannon over a keg of beer at a party on the lake. "I had an abortion today," she said, drinking from her foamy cup.

I stared at her. "Are you okay?"

She shrugged. "Yeah."

I went back over to my group of friends to gossip. "And she's *here*," I told them, "drinking *beer!*" We looked on in horror.

Dr. B injects fentanyl and Versed into the IV on Maria's right arm. "This will make you more comfortable and re-laxed, like a few cocktails," she explains to Maria, winking at me. I realize I should have done more research before com-ing into the room. On the procedure, on the meds they're using, on the exact moments Maria might need me most.

The truth is, Lauren and I have kind of been winging it since we partnered with City Hospital last week, still not believing—after months of being shut down by other clin-ics—that they actually wanted abortion doulas in this room. We've been more focused on the logistical rush: getting time off work, meeting the clinicians and counselors, figuring out how to get from one room to the next in the hospital's maze of corridors. (As we grew our organization, we would find that a combination of "winging it," just jumping the hell in with both feet, and meticulously scheduling ourselves would get us through many days.)

My background is in research and development; I've nev-er done anything that even hints at direct care. The design of this project has been strictly theoretical up to this point, mostly speaking at conferences about the model with bits and pieces of clinical intelligence from Lauren's brief stint at a birth center. The closest I've been to an abortion was sitting in the waiting room at Planned Parenthood while a friend went behind closed doors, coming out hours later no longer pregnant. Even though I had trained as a birth doula the year before, I had yet to attend a birth. And anyway, how do you prepare for something that hasn't existed in this exact form before, at least as far as we knew? What exactly was an abortion doula? What did I need to learn?

One thing I would learn is that the process of undergoing a procedure that is only five to seven minutes in length can become a complicated, jagged puzzle our clients have to put together, often in isolation. Each puzzle piece represented a decision our client would make along the way, sedation selection being only one of these pieces.

The "cocktail" metaphor Dr. B used described the sensation of the client becoming more relaxed and drowsy due to her anxiety level being reduced and her physical pain being alleviated by the medication. This sounded great to me. Who wouldn't want this to be her experience of abortion? I would just as quickly see some of the drawbacks of this type of sedation, however. The client's memory of the procedure would be negligible in many cases. For those wanting a more embodied experience of the abortion, this would be problematic. Not to mention, the more drugs used, the higher the cost in most clinics. Recovery time would also be extended and a personal escort would be required to take a client home from the abortion. Again, problematic for anyone who could not spare more time than the abortion itself required, or for people who could not or would not tell a family member or friend to meet them at the clinic after.

I wonder who Maria's support person is, who will be

taking her home from her abortion. My eyes shift back and forth between her and the foot of the bed where Dr. B is reviewing the finer points of the procedure with Dr. W, a resident who started her rotation a few weeks ago. They turn to face us. "Okay, Maria, I'm going to do a pelvic exam now. Open your legs until you feel the sides of my hands," Dr. W says gently in Spanish.

Maria winces at the pressure of the exam. *Shit, what do I do?* I quickly flash back to my birth doula training, looking for guidance. "*No, no, no, not like this. You want to hold her like this,*" my trainer had yelled. "*You need to build up the muscle in those upper arms!*" Not helpful. I shake the memory from my head. I'm unsure of how I fit into this space, surrounded by "experts." It's one of the most common feelings for any new doula until we realize we aren't supposed to be experts; our clients don't need another expert in the room.

Ann grabs Maria's hand and nods at me to do the same, sensing my panic. "Respire profundo, respire profundo," she coaches Maria and me.

"Respire," I whisper, smiling at Ann gratefully and reaching for Maria's left hand with both of mine. Much of what we would learn about compassionate care would come from observing nurses and counselors.

Maria grips my hands hard and nods, inhaling and exhaling, her eyes locked into mine. I feel breathless at the intimacy of her gaze. I have typically shied away from intimacy with strangers and loved ones alike. For most of my time on earth, I may as well have been wearing a sign around my neck with the words, "You can look, but you can't touch."

But in this moment, looking into Maria's eyes, something

clicks, and I suddenly know what to do, as though the ability to care for another person has always been inside of me, dormant. My senses heighten as I begin to tune into my role, to be in two places at once, the head of the bed and the foot of the bed. I am acutely aware of the client's every breath and the doctor's every movement.

A sheet over Maria's knees offers me only a partial view of the procedure that I would come to know by heart. Betadine, an antiseptic, is smoothed onto the vagina, vulva, the upper thighs, and abdomen with a sponge. The speculum is placed and secured, followed by an injection of lidocaine into the cervix. The tenaculum is clamped and the metal cannula is inserted in progressive sizes until the cervix is properly dilated. I find myself mesmerized by the elegance of Dr. W's motions, her wrists and fingers moving with the grace of a pianist.

Maria is groggy. She drifts in and out of consciousness, occasionally waking with quick, sharp breaths. I continue to hold her hand in mine, trying to anticipate what she might need. Dr. W selects a flexible curette, measured for Maria's current number of gestational weeks. She tests its size in Maria's cervix and attaches it to the Manual Vacuum Aspirator, a tool I had once seen on a tour of Ipas—its manufacturer—in North Carolina. Dr. W presses the buttons on the side of the MVA to release the vacuum as she moves it in 180-degree angles, an in-and-out motion, feeling for the "gritty sensation" that indicates the pregnancy has been removed. Maria's moans intensify as she shifts on the table, her uterus contracting.

"*Este es el último paso,*" Dr. W tells us. I look over at the clock. It's been less than ten minutes. I brush the perspiration from Maria's face with a tissue. Her eyes are tightly closed now as she hums through what is typically the most physically difficult part of the procedure.

"*Fin,*" the doctor says anticlimactically. She deftly removes the speculum and folds the instruments back into the sheet. Dr. B leaves the room with the products of conception.

Maria has opened her eyes, our damp hands entwined. I'm not sure if it's her sweat or mine. "*Gracias,*" she says in a tone that makes me feel as if I have just won an award, though for what I'm not exactly sure. Didn't I just stand there? Wouldn't she have been fine without me?

It would take me many more abortions, many more conversations, and hours of internal reflection to learn how profound the doula role is: how "just being there," a silent observer, bearing witness to someone else's experience and reflecting it back to them can be so much and enough. Critics and supporters alike would sometimes claim the abortion doula role to be sensational or unnecessary. They would miss the bigger point and strip the entire experience of its greater meaning.

"*De nada,*" I smile back, offering Maria the rest of the Spanish that I know.

Dr. B reenters and quietly tells Dr. W that the pregnancy has been removed completely. Maria can go to recovery now. Ann eases her into the recliner, discreetly tossing the blood-soaked plastic chuck underneath her into the wastebin.

We wave goodbye.

As a reproductive justice activist for more than a decade, I have often been asked how I got into this work, what inspired me, and why doula care? These have been tough questions to answer. For years I avoided sharing my abstinence-only background, my fear of sex, the time I publicly shamed a friend for having an abortion. I thought that if I didn't fit into a perfect activist box I would be cast out of the movement.

When I started talking, though, I learned my story was more common than I thought—maybe the most common of all stories. Most women in the United States have to confront the fear we have of our own bodies and sexuality and how we project that onto others and internalize it within ourselves. When I was growing up, no one ever spoke to me in a real way about my body or my health—not even my staunchly pro-choice, hippie parents. When I ask my parents about this now, my dad shrugs wistfully, "But I thought you weren't having sex." My mom, who has always welcomed any and every topic under the sun, simply says, "I didn't know how to talk about it." They aren't alone; most parents don't know how to talk to their kids about sex. Conversation around abortion and birth in my community was not nuanced—*there was no conversation at all.* That inane and dangerous "Lifesavers" program was the only vehicle my classmates and I had to talk about or to be close to sex. We all just wanted to explore something innate and undiscovered in ourselves.

I've stopped being ashamed of my story. Mostly. It led

me to doula work. Being a doula speaks directly to the part of myself that is complex and contradictory, and it doesn't let me hide from it. It allows me to juxtapose two opposing ideas and say these are not bad or good—they just are. It opens up a space for things to be messy, unpackaged, raw, unflinchingly human. When I work with a client, I become an activist in a way I didn't know was possible. There is no box I have to fit into.

After I witnessed that first abortion, I was on fire, more alive than I'd ever been. I felt as if I was part of some sort of historical moment. I wasn't. Abortions happen every day—more than a million people have abortions every year in the United States alone. But witnessing the care and *being part of* the care that goes into the abortion experience was something I wasn't aware of before. At least not in the way I saw at the hospital that day from the doctors and nurses, and even from myself. I wanted to tell the world about this care. I wanted to capture it in a bottle and pour it over everyone who would ever have an abortion.

This would prove to be difficult. Many cities would not see the value of abortion doula care. Many pregnant people would not have access to the kind of abortion care they wanted or needed. As we expanded our work, the privilege our clients held just by virtue of the fact that they were in New York City became clear. Here, abortion is accessible up to twenty-four weeks, Medicaid covers most procedures, and there are several options for care, from at-home medical abortion to freestanding clinic abortion to hospital-based abortion. Our clients don't encounter the restrictions on abortion that people in other states face, such as mandated waiting periods, consent requirements, or unreasonable travel barriers. Our fellow doulas around the country would struggle against these restrictions and many would be denied the opportunity to ever get into a clinic.

And yet we would find, for our clients in New York City, the emotional experience of abortion often transcends many of these legal barriers. Years later Dr. B reflects on the early days of the Doula Project:

> Mostly I remember being really grateful that you were there because patients had an enormous amount of anxiety. Even though in New York City you don't always have to walk through a thick line of protesters, I think that most people who have abortions have ambivalent feelings about it. Sometimes it's a very intense, very painful part of their lives. And having somebody to attend to emotional needs and just be there and hold their hands made a huge difference in the quality of [care]. I remember [the doulas] at the head of the bed while performing procedures and really providing a lot of comfort. And that was huge. I remember watching you guys getting so attached to these people, which . . . was really touching.

The deeply collective nature of the world we would help create within the clinic walls started to show itself to me that first week. Before we entered City Hospital we imagined ourselves as totally client focused. Birth doulas, at the time, frequently held contentious relationships with labor and delivery staff, and we were prepared for a similar experience in the clinics. Yet the impact we would have on the doctors and nurses who served our clients would become a cornerstone of our mission. Dr. B remembers, "You made a big difference for people. In addition to [the patients], as a young provider, as I was at the time, it's really nice to have validation. The group of [doulas] was so kind to us as providers. You know, abortion providers don't get that much love in the world, but we got so much love and respect from you. That was really lovely."

The Doula Project would become the most rewarding work of my life, but it would never be without its hardship or stigma. It was not work I could share with my Christian community in southern Indiana. (To this day I can count on one hand the number of times I've said the word "abortion" outside the walls of my parents' homes. Meredith and I continue to lock ourselves behind closed doors—talking in hushed tones about anything "vagina related.") The fire I felt the first days and weeks and months would burn out, and I would come to carry a certain amount of pain and dread with me. My clients would change me, how I practice care and walk through the world. The abortions, the stillbirth inductions, the adoption plans, they would move into me, and I would hold on to tiny pieces of every person I cared for.

Fellow doula and energy healer Jini Tanenhaus would later tell me, "Your chakras are closed around your heart. That's very common in this line of work. You're heart-broken." Caregiving leaves a mark. And who cares for the caregiver? Who do we *let* care for us? Though Lauren and I would often pride ourselves on being "hardcore," unsentimental to the point of detachment, deep down we also needed someone to care for us. Like many caregivers, we—as well as the doulas in the stories that follow—would struggle to allow ourselves to be vulnerable in that way, to let others see us when we were scared or tender, even as we levied that brand of care to our clients and to the world.

Maria was the first—the first client in an organization that would go on to support more than thirty-five thousand people across the spectrum of pregnancy options over the next decade.

How to Use Your Birth Doula
Training . . . and How Not to Use It

A mini chapter about how traditional birth doula care doesn't always translate to the world of full-spectrum doula care. This is a list of statements that many of us heard in our doula training that we initially tried to incorporate into our organizational model. Some of it applied, and some of it did not. This section is specifically geared toward people who want to become full-spectrum doulas.

"Doulas Serve as Advocates for Their
Clients' Needs and Wishes"

The word "advocate" turns out to be pretty loaded. "Advocating" can often be interpreted as making way for an adversarial relationship with medical staff in which the doula (or advocate) has to help the patients fight for what they need. We learned the hard way that our method of advocating to medical staff on our clients' behalf has to be gentle and pleasant and, whenever possible, is best framed as a question. Once we started working with doctors, nurses, and counselors in an abortion clinic, we were able to appreciate that sometimes the clients were offered the best that the clinic could provide, even if it wasn't always perfect. Putting pressure on the clinic to help our clients get what they ideally wanted actually put some of our colleagues in an uncomfortable position where they felt unsupported by us and unable to give the client what she was asking for—simply because it wasn't available.

That said, advocating for our clients is part of our job. But understanding *how* to effectively advocate for a client as a doula—or how to help that client advocate for herself effectively—requires patience, nuance, and a gentle approach that includes the assumption that the medical staff have good intentions. Remember, fighting or "advocating" too aggressively will (understandably) upset hospital staff, and your client may suffer the consequences.

"Always Seek to Fulfill Your Client's Requests"

This strategy can also be a great way to incite the wrath of hospital staff. We once accidentally got in between nursing staff and a midwife when a client asked for something to eat—the nurses said no, and the midwife said yes—and the result of that interaction meant that everyone was upset at us and the client.

The truth is, once your client is at the hospital, whatever part of the spectrum of pregnancy care she is there for, you have to work within the system that's in place. That's why it is best to meet your client beforehand to make sure that you are both aware of the policies of the hospital, clinic, or birthing center she has chosen for her care.

"Medical Interventions Are Overused and Unnecessary"

At the time we trained to be doulas, medical interventions such as induced labor, epidurals for pain relief, and cesarean births were at an all-time high. This high was pretty frightening, with some New York City hospitals reaching a staggering one-in-three rate of C-section deliveries, almost triple what the World Health Organization recommends.

Most birth doula trainings tend to emphasize the benefits of unmedicated vaginal or "natural" birth and offer tips to help your client navigate the discomfort of labor while also avoiding the "cascade of medical interventions." In trainings, we watch videos of people giving birth in their bathtubs, surrounded by dolphins (no, we're not exaggerating—look up the video, it will bring tears to your eyes), or in the comfort of their homes surrounded by loving partners, friends, and doulas, with candles and rose oil. Compare this to the chorus of distressed narratives of people who found their hospital birth experiences to be alienating or upsetting or who felt divorced from the experience of their labor. It's enough to make anyone staunchly invested in natural birth.

As you'll read in our stories, we can definitely attest to the reality that medical interventions are overused, sometimes with harrowing results. But soon we realized that "natural birth" requires a lot of mental and emotional investment from the client and, frankly, not everyone we worked with was in that space. Given that we started by doing stillbirths and births for people who had made adoption plans, our perspective changed from encouraging natural birth to asking, "What do you need to get through this?" We talk about medical interventions by helping clients weigh risks and benefits. And yes, a lot of our clients have wanted natural labors, and we try to help them achieve that. But it's hard to talk up the benefits of an epidural-free labor when a client is having an induced stillbirth.

"Birth Plans Are Important . . . But Not How You Might Think"

When we first started out, a lot of the births we attended were ones fraught with loss—either stillbirths or people who had made adoption plans. The births were usually in hospitals—often whatever hospitals were closest to where our clients lived.

Most doula trainings will encourage the use of "birth plans" so that the doula can have a clear understanding of the client's goals and desires during the labor and delivery. We found pretty quickly that our birth plan was an important educational tool to help our clients understand the birth process. We learned the hard way that part of helping the client to understand the birth process is helping them to confront their fears. Running away from hard topics, like finding out why a client is abjectly terrified of getting a C-section, will not serve your client well if those issues come up at the time of the birth or the procedure. Figure out a way to manage fears in advance and come up with a plan.

"Doula Work Is Intuitive (and Comes with Experience)"

Yes. This fact is both very true and very unnerving to most new doulas, whose "doula intuition" is still in the early stages of development. Be patient with yourself along the way, and keep in mind the wise words of doula Christy Hall, "Remember, you're better than nothing. You're probably better than a lot." Be transparent with your client that you're new; the intuition shines through eventually.

"Know That You Don't Know Everything"

This has continued to be relevant. "You don't know everything" is a statement that is often heard in trainings, a reminder to approach doula work with humility. The truth is that we walk a strange line between being "nonmedical providers" and "knowing a lot of accurate medical stuff."

"Always Pack a Doula Bag"

The things our clients need during labor can be radically different. We learned about the famous "doula bag" at our trainings and highly recommend bringing the following items to a birth: ice packs, hot packs, bendy straws, hair ties, essential oils, face masks, latex gloves (in case things get unexpectedly messy), tennis balls and various other massagers, snacks for both you and your client, extra socks, breath mints and a toothbrush, as well as visualization and hypnobirthing exercises.

We would also like to add the following to the birth bag repertoire: trashy magazines to read with your client—especially if she gets an epidural—ditto for nail polish, a list of local resources that can help your client get on her feet, LUNA bars in every flavor they produce, a neck pillow, cash for the hospital diner where you will invariably eat your vic-

tory meal when it's all done (our menu favorite is spanakopita and french fries).

"Doulas and Doctors Go Together Like a Fish and a Bicycle"

We were warned at our birth doula training that there would
be some antagonism between doulas and doctors when we
started. Many hospitals don't have supportive policies to fa-
cilitate a client-centered labor. Instead, birth is often treat-
ed as inherently high-risk, and it can be frustrating or even
heartbreaking for the doula to witness. To that end, many
(especially new) doulas can be a little overzealous in their
desire to "advocate" for their clients (yep, there's that word
again). It can be a mutually contentious relationship.

When we started in our first clinic, we expected to be
greeted by some skepticism, but were relieved to find out
that the doctors were our biggest champions. Our relationship to the doctors became one of the most important parts
of our work, as it enabled us to build a strong client-care
team with them.

"All Doulas Should Become Certified"

The large birth doula training organizations offer certification as a professional standard. In order to become certified,
a doula must attend a certain number of births that result
in vaginal deliveries, receive good reviews from delivery staff
and birth parents, do a take-home test or write an essay, and
complete a reading list. There are also fees and dues associated with maintaining certification status.

When we left our birth doula trainings we were prepared

to pursue certification. Later, we reevaluated those goals, and we opted to not become certified. We are clear about that with our clients. No one we've worked with has been bothered that we're not certified. Choosing certification is a personal decision, and we completely respect the many reasons why doulas choose to become certified. But we believe that it is not certification that makes a good doula.

"Running a 'Doula Business' Is the End Game"

Ha ha. Ha, ha, ha, ha, ha.

Many doula trainings emphasize "the doula business" as part of their core curriculum. That's not our story. Maybe it goes without saying that we started a nonprofit for doulas because we found out quickly that asking people for money was not our strong suit. Moreover, the New York City doula "scene" was becoming saturated with doulas, many of whom were attempting to make a living from it. More importantly, we—along with many of our doulas—feel strongly that the "activism" aspect of our work, including not asking low-income clients for money, is what drives us.

But let's be clear. Doulas as a population aren't the I percent. We don't know of any doulas who are making loads of money in their work, nor do we know any doulas who got into the work because they were looking for fame and fortune. We don't disagree that it's work that deserves to be paid—it does. It's more a question of who pays: the client, a nonprofit organization, or a larger institutional structure, like Medicaid or insurance companies.

Part 2
Doulas for Doulas

Before and After
Kat and Kim

Kat stands in the doorway and calls her client's name, "Kim?" The waiting room is packed with people, some here for STI or pregnancy results, an annual GYN exam, a colposcopy. Or, like Kim, an abortion.

Kim stands up and raises her hand, her smile a thin line. Kat walks her to the exam room, located in the back left corner of the downtown Brooklyn Planned Parenthood Clinic. She shuts the door securely and confirms Kim's last name and date of birth. "I'm your doula, Kim. I'm here to make sure you're comfortable today." Kat's low, silken voice hints of her youth spent in North Carolina. She wears her brown hair short and close to her pale face, accentuating large, expressive eyes that startle and disarm at once. "I'm not medical staff, but if you have any questions, you can ask me. If I don't know the answer, I'll help you find someone who does."

Kim looks around the room, dark eyes open wide, only half listening to Kat. She gives Kat a short nod, holding her purse protectively in front of her. Kat continues, "Let's get changed, okay? First, take off everything from the waist down. Since you're not having conscious sedation, you can keep your shirt on. Gown on and open in the back, and booties over your feet; they can be a bit tricky to get on. Your clothes can just go back in this plastic bag." Kat hands Kim a clear bag, stuffed with the gown and booties, snapped together at the top with white handles.

Kat pulls the cheerful patchwork curtain closed around Kim and waits quietly on the other side, listening to the rustling of clothes moving against the stiff paper on the procedure table. She sits on a black plastic chair tucked in the corner and stretches her long legs, turning her ankles in slow circles. She is tired, having spent the majority of her week on the cardiac unit at the hospital where she is employed as a nurse. Kat has been a doula since 2010, taking several shifts a month at Planned Parenthood's Bronx and Brooklyn sites alongside her nursing job. She has served hundreds of pregnant people, heard hundreds of stories, and been exposed to the many things that come up during and around a first trimester abortion. She knows all the motions of doula care by heart, but she never just goes through the motions.

"Okay," Kim says. "I'm ready."

Kat pushes the quilted curtain open and back against the wall. The rest of the room is revealed to her once more. There is a familiarity in these surroundings, like home, everything in its place as if she could move around with her eyes closed and find what she was looking for. Kim stands next to the light pink procedure table. To her right is the nurse's computer, where stats will be tracked throughout the abortion, and a supply table is an arm's length away, over-flowing with gauze, flushes, needles and syringes of various sizes, bandages, cotton balls, tape, and tourniquets.

Across from Kim is the doctor's computer, keeper of the clients' medical records and the room's source of music, a Pandora station playing Michael Jackson. When the doctor swivels on her stool away from the computer, she will find her tool cart, prepped meticulously by the medical assistant. Beside the cart is the electric vacuum aspiration machine, a common instrument of pregnancy removal that uses an electric pump instead of a manual one and makes a louder noise than the manual vacuum aspirator. A blood pressure machine rests near the head of the procedure table, cords gathered into the basket hanging from its side. There is one frosted window and a swinging door that leads to the scrub room. When Kim lies down, she will look up and see Kat's favorite detail of the room, a ceiling light fixture that looks like the sky.

Planned Parenthood is a freestanding clinic, which means it operates outside of a hospital setting. Freestanding clinics can be public or private establishments, and because they are not connected to a hospital, they typically refer any clients with medical issues to hospital-based abortion services. They are often subjected to more antichoice protesting than a hospital-based setting would be and are also more likely to be affected by Targeted Regulation of Abortion Providers (TRAP) laws. In New York City, while there are regular groups of protesters at several clinic sites, the occurrence is much less common, as are TRAP laws. Freestanding clinics tend to be less bureaucratic than hospital-based clinics, and procedures can frequently happen the day of consultation in states where no other restrictions apply.

Kat straightens the blue-and-white chuck on the procedure table as Kim self-consciously clutches the opening gap on the back of her gown and climbs on. Kat drapes a blue sheet over her legs, covering her nakedness. Kim plays awkwardly with the booties, trying to open them. "How do these . . . ?"

"You just wanna pull the front tip over the toe and the back over the heel so they cover the bottom of your foot, like this," Kat shows her. Kim is wearing black-and-white knit stockings that reach nearly to her crotch. "These are amazing," Kat says.

"Thank you," Kim gives her a hesitant smile. She is not ready for small talk. Kat rolls the doctor's stool over and sits down so they are at eye level, a doula move meant to reduce the power level. She reflects on the interaction today, "One of the most valuable things about [our role] is the one-on-one time with the client previous [to the procedure]. Because they have that reference point, they know who we are and that we are gonna be there the whole time. Because we've *told* them we're gonna be there the whole time."

"How are you?" Kat asks.

Kim shrugs, "Okay."

"Do you have any questions?"

Kim exhales, looks up at the ceiling then back at Kat. "Is it gonna hurt?"

Kat pauses. This is one of the most common questions a

doula gets asked before a procedure. It's covered extensively in training, and while every doula has a slightly different turn of phrase, there is a standard approach that the Doula Project and the clinics we work with use. "Do you get cramps with your period?"

Since Kim is receiving only a local sedation, her experience of discomfort may be increased. Local sedation means that no medication outside of an injection of lidocaine into the cervix will be used, so the pain from cramping in the uterus is hard to avoid. Some of our clients prefer local sedation because it is cheaper, does not require a family member or friend to escort them home afterward, has minimal to no side effects, and allows them to be alert and aware of their bodies during the procedure.

"Yeah, pretty bad ones," Kim replies.

"You will feel something," Kat explains, carefully choosing her words. "Everyone has a different reaction, but for a few minutes it will feel like very strong period cramps. The good news is when that happens, it means the uterus is going back to its prepregnancy size, which is what we want." She speaks with her hands but not in an affected way, more as if her long, thin fingers are doing a slow dance. Each word is intentional, punctuated by pauses in the middle of a statement—a chance to collect her thoughts. Kim's hands clench tighter around the sheet at Kat's explanation. "How are you feeling?" Kat asks gently, breaking from her semi-prepared remarks.

"I guess I thought I wasn't going to feel anything," Kim says, searching Kat's face.

"Kim, you can do it. The procedure is very fast, usually less than five minutes, and you're in really good hands. Your doctor and nurse and medical assistant are great. We're gonna help you. You're gonna be fine." Even after having this conversation a hundred times before, Kat feels an ache for her client. She knows that these words don't always alleviate the anxiety or lessen the dread of what is to come. But she has made a vow to never lie about a procedure, to never pretend that her client won't feel anything.

It's often difficult as a doula to answer certain questions. There are some that always hit you at your core, and they are often the ones on many of our clients' minds:

Will it hurt?

Will I be able to get pregnant again?

What do they do with the baby?

Do you think God will forgive me?

And then the question that tends to throw most doulas off, no matter how often it is asked: *Have you ever had an abortion?*

Clients might ask this question because they think if you have had an abortion, you will know firsthand about the pain, or you will be more accepting of their being there, or you will understand more what they are going through emotionally. In many ways, a client asking this question speaks to the more equal space doulas hold with them than, say, doctors or nurses; rarely do clients ever ask them about their abortions.

Doulas decide for themselves if they want to disclose personal information about their own reproductive health to their clients and what end it will serve. Several doulas, including Kat, have been drawn to this work because of their own abortion experiences.

In November 2006, Kat was living just outside of Washington, DC, in Silver Spring, Maryland. She had finished graduate school a few years before and decided to stick around the area. Her American Studies degree was burning a hole in her pocket. She hadn't found any employer too impressed with it, so she was working at a bookstore, which paid a few bills but offered little inspiration. She had just gotten back together with her ex, a cook who worked at the local chili joint and wore dreadlocks tied off with glass beads. They had sex in his basement apartment, her first time in many months. Each breath she took was filled with the cat litter that festered in the corner, the stale pot smoke that clung to the air.

A few weeks later, she and her sister went to visit their grandma in Tennessee. Kat woke to a beautiful, cloudless day, but she was worried. She had missed her period. She took her grandma's car to the grocery store down the street and bought a pregnancy test. To her surprise, it came up negative. "I don't believe it," she told her sister, coming out of the bathroom.

"Okay, so say you *are* pregnant," her sister posed. "What will you do?"

"I don't know . . . I think I might keep it."

When she got back to her apartment in Maryland later that week, she took another test, this time in the morning.

The two lines were so faint, she couldn't be sure it was positive. She made a doctor's appointment.

"Well, what are you gonna do?" the doctor asked while taking her blood. Kat narrowed her eyes. *Do not ask me that now.* By the end of that weekend, the official test had come back positive. Kat was pregnant.

The days and weeks that followed were a bone-chilling, mid-Atlantic gray. She immediately felt nauseous, a condition that would last throughout her pregnancy. She wanted someone else to tell her what to do. She started calling clinics and obstetricians, seeing what her options were. She stopped smoking pot.

She went to her boyfriend's house one night to share the news. They sat side by side on his bed, hunched under the low ceilings. She turned to face him. "I'm pregnant."

Without looking at her, he shot across the small room, as far away as he could get from her, and busied himself lighting incense. After some time passed, he spoke. "If you want to keep it, we can be a family."

Like so many women, Kat's life circumstances at the time would ultimately move her toward an abortion. "Nothing about my life would sustain being a mom," she says now. "I was like, 'This is not the kind of family I want.' In the back of my head I knew I was gay and needed to come out eventually. 'If I have a kid right now, what?' I definitely didn't *want* to do it. I was heartbroken about it and real fucked up, real fucked up . . . for a while."

For the next two weeks, Kat and her boyfriend barely spoke. Kat's nausea kept her on a diet of saltine crackers and

Subway sandwiches, anything bland she could keep down. She tried every antinausea medication she could find and even bought an armband that triggered specific pressure points. She still wound up pulling her car to the side of the road to puke yellow bile. She started using marijuana again to soothe the nausea, numb the emotional pain. But part of her was still considering keeping the pregnancy.

One day, on her way to pick up a friend from the airport, Kat was confronted by a pro-life poster campaign: *Scared? Pregnant? We are here.*

"I don't know what to do," she said on the drive home.

"It sounds to me like you know what you want to do," her friend responded gently.

"What? What do I want to do?" Kat was still looking for a way around making this decision.

"Kat . . . I'm not gonna tell you."

Kat stared straight ahead.

Later that week, she called a Baltimore abortion clinic and made an appointment. The DC clinic was notorious for its protesters, and Kat didn't want to deal with that on top of everything else. By this time it was the holidays, and her procedure wouldn't be scheduled until late December. That Christmas Eve Kat found herself alone. Her roommates and friends had left town. She hadn't heard from her boyfriend in days. She fell asleep on her roommate's bed in front of the television, waking up to a miserable, dark sky. She considered spending Christmas Day on her own, heartache and sitcoms her sole companions.

Instead, she called a couple that was spending the holiday

in town. They told her to come over. When Kat arrived, she found piles of presents wrapped with her name on them. Her friends had scrounged around their home, looking for special trinkets to give her. Her abortion faded to the back of her mind for one sweet night.

The doctor enters through the swinging door of the scrub room, nurse and medical assistant closely behind. "Hi, Kim. How are you?"

An experienced doula knows that this is a major shift for a client, the moment the process becomes real. No matter the rapport a doula has built, anxiety usually increases the moment medical staff comes in. Clients know it's a signal the procedure is about to start. Kat notices Kim tense up considerably, her legs tightening together on the table. *This is it,* that tightening says. *This is it—here we go.*

Kim regains her composure quickly, hands interlaced tensely in her lap. She smiles and says a shy "Hello."

"Do you have any questions for me, Kim?" The doctors at Planned Parenthood always make sure to say the patient's name, a technique meant to individualize the experience.

"Umm . . . I don't think so . . ." She glances at Kat, who raises her eyebrows and smiles encouragingly. Often Kat will help a client ask the doctor a question, if needed. She recognizes the heightened emotion in the room and tries to help trigger her clients' memories about anything they want to speak to the doctor about. This is a key aspect of the doula role: building that relationship before medical staff enters, explaining in advance who all the medical staff are and how many people will be in the room, helping clients advocate for themselves when they feel nervous or intimidated. "I'm good," Kim finishes.

"So, we will be placing an IUD after the procedure today, right?" the doctor confirms with Kim, who nods her assent to inserting the long-acting contraceptive while her cervix is dilated. "Everything is going to go great. The procedure is quick and safe."

They reset Kim at the table, lifting her hips so the chuck can be repositioned. Her hips are then lowered, with her butt way down to the bottom of the table and her feet in stirrups. Kat takes her position at the top of the table, her hand resting near Kim's shoulders.

"Okay, Kim, we're going to begin," says the doctor, checking her position. "I just want to ask again and see if you have any questions."

"No," she says and lays her head back against the table with a long exhale as the doctor's gloves go on. Kim looks up at the ceiling and smiles at the light cover decorated with clouds and bluebells. "That's nice," she says.

"Isn't it?" says Kat.

"It's nice to see something pretty here. It's nice to have something pretty to look at." Kim says, and Kat nods in agreement.

"Let your legs fall open until you feel the back of my hands," the doctor says. Kim is still nervous, but as the doctor begins her manual exam of Kim's pelvis, something Kim is familiar with from previous visits to the gynecologist, she relaxes a little. Things are finally underway.

Kat goes back to Kim's striped stockings, "So where did you get these great socks?"

"I actually made them myself," Kim says, clearly proud.

"Are you serious?" The whole room makes sounds of exclamation. Kim says she is a fashion designer, taking classes at the Fashion Institute of Technology and hoping to go to Parsons. Her eyes find Kat's as the doctor places the speculum.

A few days before her abortion, Kat stepped outside her house and found an envelope addressed to her, filled with cash and those familiar glass beads. *What the hell?* It could only be from one person: her boyfriend had cut off his dreadlocks in some bizarre grand gesture and left her money to pay for the abortion. She was furious and asked her roommate to take her to the clinic instead. She didn't want to deal with him.

It was the perfect day to get an abortion: ugly, gray, cold but not too cold. Kat was still sick, nauseated and miserable, unsure of her decision up until the last second. Her uncertainty had nothing to do with her religious beliefs. It was more that she was in her late twenties and thought that maybe this was her only chance to have a kid. And in spite of herself, she still wanted to make it work with her boyfriend. He showed up at the clinic and sat with her roommate in the waiting room while Kat went through the processing and paperwork, the precounseling, and the ultrasound.

During her ultrasound the doctor angled the monitor toward her so it was directly in her line of vision. "I have a retroverted uterus, and they had to use [the ultrasound]," she remembers. "It was sitting right there in front of me, and they were not thoughtful enough to turn it away. And I was gonna look because I wanted to hurt more."

Afterward she went to the smaller waiting room to sit with the other patients, longing for someone to talk to. She watched *Dr. Dolittle* two times in a row before they called her to the room where her abortion would take place. The procedure was physically painful, but she was more focused on the ultrasound. It was back, glowing through the dim lights in the room. She gritted her teeth and didn't cry. When the procedure was finished she looked at her empty uterus reflected back at her in the monitor.

The nurses in recovery were nice. Kat cried a little and felt immediate relief. On the ride home she lay down in the back seat of the car. *I should feel worse than this.* But she was just so glad the nausea was gone. Days later she would draw two pictures of her uterus, one with a fetus and one without.

"It's not that there are no days that I'm haunted by my abortion," Kat says now. "But it's so completely different, that part of my emotional life. I don't think I would've healed from that in the same way if I hadn't been part of the Doula Project. When I started with the Doula Project, it was at least four years after the abortion, and I was not healed from it. And being part of the project . . . in some ways it was salve on a wound. I didn't notice it, and then I realized I can talk about [my abortion] and not cry . . . this is what healed me, I have no doubt."

Kat maneuvers the purple recliner clumsily through the hallway, attempting a sharp right turn into the recovery room. She passes her co-doula bringing another client into the procedure room next door. She briefly wonders what this coworker is like as a doula: if she smoothes back her client's hair, counts through the pain, holds the same quiet space. There are few opportunities to see other doulas in action during abortions. Kat's own style has changed through the years.

When she started out, she was terrified. "You take emotional hits in the beginning. It's so easy for me to sit here five years in and be cool as a cucumber about it. I was rocked after my first few shifts. I was like, 'What just happened?' It's intense. Civilians don't understand, your partners aren't going to understand, your best friends aren't going to understand. They might listen to you, but they don't get it."

Even with the best training it's impossible to predict exactly what each procedure will be like, how a client will respond, and what the staff will need from you. Many doulas have no medical background at all and have only seen an operating room on television or visited labor and delivery after a friend gives birth. This is often the first time they have practiced direct care in general; it is usually their political ideology or the desire to connect with people on the ground that has led them to the work. They face the utter insecurity of feeling like they don't know what to do: how to engage their clients, where to stand, when to offer a comforting touch—the things that seem simple and unthinking to the seasoned doula but initially elude them.

Over time Kat has learned some tricks: how to read the energy in the room, the tone of her client's voice, her client's body language. Whenever she does feel lost in the work or unsure of how to be, she thinks back to a meditation that fellow doula Jini Tanenhaus read during her training when she was first becoming an abortion doula. Kat tries to be what Jini taught her to be—a calming presence. "We imagined a living creature that we loved uncomplicatedly and let that fill the space around us. That is what I try to do."

Even as Kat has gotten comfortable in her role, she has questioned her place in the room as a middle class white woman. She has wondered "if we should be doing this work as mostly middle class white women who serve brown and black women . . . what right do we have?" She reflects, "I also think that it is valuable work. I've just seen it make a difference for a lot of people. And they walk away, and they go live their lives, and they don't need me to hold their hands. But support is support, and I've had too many people be like, 'I'm so glad you were there.' And for me to act like it doesn't matter that I was there belittles their appreciation."

Kat wheels Kim's chair into an empty space along the back wall, next to three other large reclining chairs. That morning she had laid blue chucks on the floor to catch the water spitting out of the radiator. Sunlight shines in through frosted windows that reach up to high ceilings, their molding creating a frame for the room. Even though it's winter, the windows are open, offering relief from the simmering heating system.

Gloria, the recovery nurse, sits at her desk along the wall

adjacent to the recliners. She is a revered institution at the clinic and has spent more than forty years supporting patients after abortions, having begun her work before *Roe v. Wade*. The doulas have built a sort of cult following around her, frequently exchanging "Gloria Stories" and comparing presents she brings them each week: a flowered makeup bag, a pastel cell phone stand, a new plastic water bottle, a ceramic coffee mug. Once she saved a magazine clipping of an actress that reminded her of one of the doulas, carrying it with her for weeks until the doula arrived for shift.

Gloria rushes over to Kim, her sneakers a size too big and squeaking on the floor. "Push back, push back in the chair," she tells Kim gruffly, pulling at the head of the recliner. Its base pops out, lifting Kim's legs. Kat wraps the blood pressure cuff around Kim's arm and pumps, recording her stats on a Post-it she will hand to Gloria. Kat then approaches the station opposite the recliners, rinsing her hands in the sink and putting on gloves, pouring ginger ale into a small plastic cup, and grabbing a few packets of saltines. She empties two ibuprofens into a second cup, handing everything one by one to Kim.

Downtown Brooklyn honks and shouts through the cracked windows. Gloria has the television on, lately tuned to *Jeopardy* reruns, *One Life to Live*, and *All My Children*. She is now hunched near another patient, giving discharge instructions. "Wait to eat something until you get home . . ."

Kim is tired and cramping. Kat snaps open a hot pack and shakes it until she feels heat. She sits in the empty recliner next to Kim and hands her the hot pack. Kim places it on her abdomen. The air is heavy with disinfectant spray. They don't say much.

"How long do I have to wait?" Kim asks after a while.

"Not too long, probably," Kat says. "The recovery room nurse will give you some instructions and make sure you're stable. Then you can get changed."

Kim nods and looks at her phone.

"Is someone waiting for you?" Kat asks.

"Yeah," she says. "My boyfriend is in the waiting room."

"Is he being supportive?" Kat asks.

Kim sighs. "He is, but he kinda wanted me to keep it. But he understands it's just not time yet. I want to finish school. He's in school too, so he understands, but"—she begins to cry—"it's just sad."

Kat hands her a tissue, "It's totally normal to be sad and have feelings about what you've just been through."

"Does everyone cry?" Kim asks.

"Everyone has a different reaction," Kat responds. "But it's not easy for anyone. No one wants to have an abortion."

Kim is quiet. "Thank you for being there," she says, sniffling. "That made it easier."

"You're so welcome," Kat says. "I'm so glad I could be here."

They continue to watch *Jeopardy*. Gloria comes over to check Kim's bleeding and review discharge instructions. Gloria then guides her to the changing area and pulls the curtain closed. When Kim emerges moments later, Kat stands up and walks with her down the long hallway to the main waiting room.

"How are you feeling?" Kat asks.

"Better," she says. "I feel better."

"You look better," Kat tells her.

They reach the door, and Kat wishes her good luck with school and her career. "I'll be looking for you in the magazines."

Kim laughs and hugs Kat. "Thank you."

"Take good care of yourself." Kat holds open the door.

"I will."

Kat heads back to recovery to gather her things, grabbing her purse, jacket, and the flowered cloth grocery bag from Gloria. It was a good day. Even though she had been reluctant to come in that morning, as she sometimes is, she feels rejuvenated by the clients she met and by her bond with the clinic staff. After all these years, she can't really imagine herself leaving this work.

"There aren't a lot of places in my life where I feel like my presence makes a difference," Kat says now, pausing. "I was raised to feel like the world was indifferent to my presence. I've gotten over a lot of that, but at base I kind of feel like 'okay if you're here, okay if you aren't.' But as a doula I feel like . . . because I have been told so many times by so many clients that my presence is important to them, that my presence made a difference to their experience . . ." She shrugs. "I've never felt more like anything than a doula, I've never felt more like 'this is just what I am'."

Here for You, Here for Me
Kira and Lauren

Kira eyes the overflowing shelf of potato chips, determining which flavor might couple best with the cookie-dough ice cream she plans to use as a dip. The sour cream and onion from the day before was good, but she wants to try something new. This is her third trip to the drugstore this week, and she is committed to getting the combination right.

It feels good to be out of her apartment, clearheaded for the first time in months. Her blue eyes are beginning to shine bright again.

Barbecue?

She frowns. She doesn't even like barbecue chips.

Her arms fall to her sides, the pint of ice cream precarious in her fingers. "Holy shit," she says aloud, her voice flat.

"I didn't need a pregnancy test for confirmation, because I knew," Kira remembers today. But she mechanically picks out the bag of barbecue chips, rearranging the items in her arms, and walks slowly toward the back of the store. She searches the signs that hang over each aisle until she reaches the pregnancy tests. She selects one at random, bringing it to the register, absently handing money to the cashier before stepping out into the October evening. The cheap plastic bag holding her purchases blows in the breeze.

Her apartment is seven blocks from the drugstore. *I have seven blocks to figure out what I'm going to do.* She sets out down the street, walking through the commercial district of Astoria as it turns tree-lined and residential. Of course, she is going to terminate. That much she is sure of. It's more a question of whom she will call first, who will be her doula, which doctor she will request to perform her abortion. Most importantly, is she going to tell Jay?

Back when she and Jay were in a relationship, they had a conversation about this very moment. "If you get pregnant, please tell me. Even if we aren't together," he had said.

"I don't know if I would, if I were terminating," she had replied.

"No, please. Tell me."

But everything is different now. So much has happened between them. They haven't even spoken in two months. Does his plea still stand?

Kira walks through the front door of her small one bed-room, turns into the living room, and dumps the contents of the bag onto the ottoman. She sinks back into the couch, opening the barbecue chips and eating them one at a time. She stares at the pregnancy test.

Pregnancy had been the last thing on her mind. She has the NuvaRing. She and her psychiatrist even came up with a foolproof plan: *Keep one in at all times; skip your period. That way you never forget.* Besides, she isn't having sex, and hasn't slept with Jay since they got back from Ecuador in . . . early August? Her memory is a little fuzzy. Of course, she has noticed her body changing, that her appetite is coming back. After a summer of almost no food, weight gain has been a relief, a sign that she is finally healthy, finally becoming herself again.

Suddenly, Kira's thoughts are interrupted by the taste of bile mixing with the powdery barbecue. She jumps up from the couch, pushing through the kitchen to the bathroom. Throwing open the toilet seat, she heaves out the chips. She raises her head and wipes her mouth. Now that she thinks about it, she has been throwing up a lot lately, most recently at a Doula Project leadership meeting at Curly's in the East Village. She had bolted from the diner table packed with her doula friends and mostly missed the toilet, her vomit landing on the cracked floor and yellow walls of the airless bathroom.

It's time. Kira picks up the pregnancy test from the ottoman, returns to the toilet, unwraps the stick, and pees on it. She places it on the lid of the trash can. The instructions on the test say to wait three minutes for the results, but two perfect dark pink lines show up immediately.

She remains seated on the toilet and positions the second test underneath her. Same result. Today, she reflects, "I kick myself because I wish I would've kept one. Part of me wants to remember every detail of this time. And not because I feel good about it, but because it was such an important time in my life."

Kira enters her bedroom and picks up her phone, her mind racing. *It's Tuesday. You know procedures are on Tuesdays, Thursdays, and Fridays, and you want Dr. A to do this procedure. You need to find out if she works these days. You need to call Lauren immediately.*

"I'm pregnant," she says when Lauren answers.

After a pause, Lauren asks, "How do you feel about that?"

Kira blinks at the sunset through the window in her bedroom. Somehow it's still light outside. "I'm going to have an abortion."

"Do you know how far along you are?"

"I have . . . no idea," Kira replies. She knows they can't schedule a procedure until they determine how many weeks pregnant she is. While Lauren figures out the logistics for an ultrasound the next day, Kira can't take her eyes off her body: her abdomen is hard, her breasts large and swollen. It all makes so much sense. *You're fucking pregnant right now.*

After she hangs up with Lauren, she calls her coworker and closest friend Laura, who will accompany her to her procedure later in the week. "I'm not going to be at work tomorrow. I'm pregnant."

Finally, she calls Jay and leaves a message. "You need to call me back as soon as possible. I need to speak with you immediately."

Her phone rings a few minutes later.

"Are you safe?" Jay asks seriously. "Is everything okay?"

"No. You need to come over now."

Twenty minutes later he is at her door. She brings him into the living room where they sit rigidly next to each other on the edge of the couch cushions.

"I'm telling you because I made you this promise," she begins. "I don't need anything from you, but I'm pregnant."

He looks at her without comment.

"Do you want to touch my abdomen?" she asks after a while.

"No," he says quietly.

Kira arrives at City Hospital the next morning for her ultrasound. She rides the elevator to the fourth floor of the outpatient clinic and steps onto the sun-dappled floor. A massive skylight casts a warm glow over the women's health patients scattered throughout the waiting area. She pauses to get her bearings. She feels anxious about the day but grateful for her knowledge of the process through her work as an abortion doula.

A few years before, Kira was working at a women's foundation in New York City when an email appeared in her inbox that read, "Apply to be an Abortion Doula!" She filled out an application immediately. Her previous job had been in direct care, and she missed the one-on-one connection, the intense intimacy. She had heard about birth doulas, but it never interested her. Abortion doulas were a totally new concept; it felt like the missing link in her life. "I had no idea what I was getting myself into and no idea how impactful [the Doula Project] would be for me. And I had no idea how much I would love it." By the time that she came in for her own ultrasound, she had already attended hundreds of abortions, sat on the leadership circle of the organization, and managed a clinic site in Queens.

Kira is buzzed through the clinic doors and greeted by

Lauren, who is both a doula and a clinical coordinator at City Hospital. She takes Kira to an exam room to meet her ultrasound tech. The tech explains the exam and shows her the instrument for the transvaginal ultrasound. It is a sleek wand that will be placed inside her to reproduce her pregnancy on screen.

"Can I see the screen?" Kira asks, rising on her elbows from the head of the bed, her body full with pregnancy and wand.

"Are you sure?" the tech asks.

"I'm so curious."

The tech turns the screen toward her. Kira has seen dozens of ultrasounds before. She is familiar with the grainy black-and-white images they produce, the way your eyes have to squint and adjust to locate the pregnancy. She discovers she is ten-and-a-half weeks along, the pregnancy only a little larger than a lima bean. The tech points it out on the monitor, "Right there."

Kira's eyes well with tears she didn't even know she was holding back. She can't stop looking. Formations of tiny legs and tiny arms lighten the screen. *That's my baby.* The weight of her decision hits her. The life that she planned with Jay is captured in this image. The wedding they talked about, the children they would raise together, the family they would become. It was the life Kira had been looking for.

But as their relationship progressed, cracks started to show. Then those cracks turned into deep fractures. Kira was overcome by work stress and felt herself sinking into depression, something she had battled in the past. Jay decided to leave for Ecuador at that time to volunteer in a health clinic, leaving Kira without word from him for more than a month. By the time they reunited, she had tried many different medications that had turned her mind and body inside out. Jay simply told her, "I don't want this for the rest of my life," and walked out.

Kira had not anticipated her reaction to the ultrasound, her intense connection to the pregnancy. As she leaves the clinic, she realizes that her activism and years as an abortion doula could never have prepared her for her own emotional response. She could never have known what it was like to be pregnant.

As Kira reaches out to friends and colleagues in the field, she also finds herself unprepared for the response she gets from a movement she cares so much about. Words and phrases that are part of Kira's vocabulary as a doula: "You'll get through this," "Products of conception," and "Parasite" make her feel distanced from the work she has dedicated her life to. She knows everyone is only trying to be supportive, but they seem to be missing the point—calling her pregnancy everything but "baby" feels wrong and awful to her. *No! This is the life I planned!*

When Kira talks about this now she still feels angry:

I had identified with this political movement that felt like home to me. Fighting for people's choices. And the language we were using—it made me feel like I was being separated from my own experience, like I had to separate my politics from my experience when it was all the same.

We say "mirror the language of your client," but there was an assumption that because I was so political and had done all this work that I wouldn't feel anything about it.

When she speaks to her friends about it, they shift their responses. They admit they are unaware of what she needs and how she is feeling. But she still remembers those initial words and their connection to the larger pro-choice framework that many doulas and activists are trained on. Now, Kira says:

> I still don't think we get it right. There are plenty of times now that people say, "It's just a medical procedure." No, it's not having your tonsils out. It's not having your wisdom teeth pulled. You're having life pulled from your body. And that's not to say that I regret my decision. That's not at all what I'm saying. It's just that I don't think we are doing a service to people by taking the emotion out of abortion as a means of making it legal and right and just and slapping a term of "medical procedure" on it. It erases the story. The procedure itself is five to seven minutes. But there is a lifetime that happened before that.

The evening before her abortion, Kira walks to her neighborhood nail salon for a pedicure. She wants everything from the waist down to be manicured, clean, pretty. The medical staffers that will ask her tomorrow to remove her underwear and place her feet into stirrups are—in many ways—her colleagues.

Once at the salon she climbs into the oversized recliner,

her pants tightening as she sits, her tank top revealing her small belly. The nail technician points at it. Kira nods. "I am pregnant," she verifies, which gets her a big smile. She doesn't mention she is having an abortion in twelve hours.

She returns home, freshly painted, and scrubs and shaves her vulva. She orders two takeout meals, one for that night and one for tomorrow after her abortion. At 11:30 p.m., she picks up her phone to text Lauren. She wants to write, *"Don't forget about me. I'm coming in tomorrow morning. Don't be sick, don't let any other doula be there—I don't want them to know."* Instead, she sends, *"Am I making the right decision?"*

Lauren responds immediately. *"You would make a wonderful mother, and it's okay that now is not the right time. You help so many other people, and it's okay to focus on you."* Kira lets those words take her into a deep sleep.

She had planned to take a cab to the hospital the next day. Instead, she wakes up early and well rested, so she hops on the N train, arriving at City Hospital two hours before her appointment. Around 6:00 a.m. she enters the general surgery waiting room. She wants to make sure she gets the perfect seat so she can be aware of everything happening around her.

Despite having supportive people in her life and knowing that she would have someone with her during the procedure, she remembers feeling frightened and alone:

> I recognize my experience is different than a lot of our clients. Because I handpicked my doula, and my doula was a very dear friend of mine, I was able to meet my doula

long before I had my procedure. But I was terrified. Actually terrified. Because I knew too much. I had way too much information about the procedure and what led up to it. The anticipation in our clients' eyes when they sit in the waiting room . . . the waiting was the thing I was really nervous about.

There are about forty-five chairs to choose from. First, she tries the far corner but feels trapped. She skips past the wall near the entrance—she doesn't want her back to the door. She chooses a seat squarely in the middle of the room and watches as people begin to drift in. *Are they having abortions?* she wonders. *Is she alone too?* She checks her phone over and over for texts from Lauren and Laura.

Laura arrives fifteen minutes later. "I knew you would be here early," she says. Both of their hands tremble as they reach for each other.

At 8:00 a.m. a nurse walks into the room, calling names one by one.

"Kira Laffe."

She joins a line of women outside the door. *Everyone knows we're having abortions,* she thinks. They are led down the hall to another, smaller waiting room. They are handed white cloth gowns and blue booties and ushered all together into the changing area. Everyone hurriedly removes their clothes and throws their belongings into lockers, eyes and heads down. "Your phone too," says the nurse.

Kira sits down in the waiting room, for once relieved she doesn't know Spanish like the other women. She doesn't want to talk to anyone. But her phone was her last link to the outside world, to Lauren. *Where is she? She's gonna forget me; she's gonna forget me.* Kira had asked to be the first procedure of the day, another privilege of being a doula. She starts to worry that Lauren will miss it. Her whole body feels cold and clammy, slick with sweat. She sits wringing her hands, peeling the hangnails from her fingers until blood pools, the same color as the polish she had carefully picked the night before.

"Kira Laffe." The resident doctor is standing in the doorway.

Kira gets up and shuffles toward her, out of the room. She looks down at her booties, the bottom of her gown trembling with the shake of her entire body.

Oh my God, I can't go yet. Lauren isn't here.

As she is about to enter the procedure room, she looks up and sees Lauren running toward her down the long hallway. She throws her arms around Kira.

"I thought you forgot about me," Kira says.

Lauren swats at Kira's shoulder. "Of course not."

The procedure room is filled with people: the attending doctor, a resident, a nurse, and med students. Kira lies on the cold table, waiting to be injected with the medication that induces moderate sedation. "When the meds started to go through, I don't know if it was that or the fear itself," she recalls, "but as soon as I lay back, the magnitude of the situation struck me." She remembers realizing that she had been afraid of Lauren not being there: "I knew from being in those procedures, while there was an attempt to make a connection with a patient, they had a limited amount of time and almost a desensitization to the emotional aspect. And I get it, and I don't think it's every provider . . . but I was terrified that I was going to be left alone with the noises in the room."

Kira and Lauren had never been touchy-feely other than the occasional hug at greeting. And like most doulas in the Project, Kira had never seen Lauren in action. Typically only doulas who served as trainers were privy to another doula's work, and Lauren and Kira operated out of different clinics. Kira knows there is nothing anyone can say to make her feel better. She herself is incapable of talking. All she wants is a grounding touch, someone to steady her physically.

Kira clutches her gown with her right hand as she waits for the procedure to begin, and Lauren takes hold of her left, placing it between her two hands on top of Kira's body. It is exactly what she needs; Kira immediately feels comforted. Very few words pass between them throughout the procedure. Kira searches Lauren's eyes, looking for information. Lauren looks back with no fear or trepidation. Kira begins to cry.

Lauren takes one hand to brush the first tear away and then lets them come. She smooths back Kira's hair. "It's okay to close your eyes. You're safe."

Kira dozes off, waking up at the end of the procedure to the pressure from a uterine massage. She reaches down, attempting to push Dr. A's hands away. Lauren takes Kira's hands and places them back in her lap while the doctor finishes.

Kira closes her eyes again and wakes up, disoriented, in the recovery room. A nurse she hasn't seen before has her arm and is attaching a blood-pressure cuff. She hands Kira a saltine cracker that Kira places in her dry mouth. She is too tired to chew and lets it sit on her tongue as she stares at the nurse.

"Here are your clothes," the nurse says. "Time to go home."

Kira goes into the changing room and puts on her pants and bra. She studies herself in the mirror. *Why didn't you just wait another week so you could feel what it would be like to be pregnant just a little longer?*

There is a knock at the door. Kira opens it to find Lauren holding a huge cupcake in both hands. "For you." They hug, and Lauren promises to check in later. Kira closes the door again and rests her hand on her abdomen. It's over.

"It was really perfect," she recalls. "I can't imagine going through that without a doula. If I hadn't known what doulas were, could I have done it? Of course, so many women do. But I would've felt so alone. To this day, I don't really know what to do about the guilt I feel about not remembering everything. I feel like I owe it to myself to remember. So to have someone there who does remember it and is willing to talk to me about it over and over and over and over is so special to me."

Kira has a doula shift scheduled shortly after her own procedure. The day she is due back in the clinic, Lauren asks, "Are you sure you're ready to do this? Are you sure you *want* to do this?"

"I'm more ready to do this than I'm ready to go back to living life normally."

Kira wasn't sure if her own abortion would change her as a doula, make her different, better, more connected to her clients. In a way, before her termination she had carried some amount of guilt and insecurity, having never experienced a termination yet guiding others through it. And now, though she knows you can't really understand what it's like without having one yourself, she finds her own caregiving methods as a doula are not so different. "I thought it might be, but . . . I think the doulas do an amazing job explaining the procedure, usually better than the doctors do, talking about pain. And I don't think it has to do with personal experience. I think it comes from witnessing it. And so did I feel like a different doula? No."

Kira says that the only thing that was different was that when someone asked if she'd had an abortion, the answer was yes. She says that in some situations, she would share that information without being asked, especially if a client said, "What kind of person does this?" She wanted to create a space to convey that "lots of us do."

Walking Gracefully through
an Operating Room

Whitney and Shelly

Whitney finds a corner in City Hospital's freezing operating room (OR) and waits for her client to roll in on a hospital bed. She holds herself tall and poised, by this point used to the circus that is the operating room. After a year of working here as an abortion doula, she is both inured to and disoriented by this strange chaotic place—the tension between eminence and nothingness, anticipation and dire urgency.

She feels a little awkward during these intermissions. Her only purpose is to be the doula for the people having procedures today; she doesn't have much to do until her client comes down. She puts on her game face, the one that appears open and warm, and she fakes it until she makes it. If Whitney doesn't tell you that she feels a little shy and that sometimes she isn't sure she knows what she's doing, you would never know. Her friendliness shines through first as she says, "I can talk to a door knob—I can really talk."

Like many doulas in the Doula Project, Whitney finds

herself simultaneously drawn to working in the OR and utterly alienated by it. She began attending second trimester abortions about a year after she trained with the Doula Project. It was initially challenging for her to make the jump from "training" to "doing." A month after the training she became pregnant and had a first trimester abortion at City Hospital. It was an unflinchingly intimate look at the healthcare system and the benefit of having a doula during an abortion. Lauren was able to attend. After, Whitney needed time to think about whether she was ready to work with the Doula Project or if it would provoke stress or too many negative feelings. She began by working with clients who were having second trimester abortions, an entirely different kind of procedure that happens in a physically different place in the hospital from where she had her abortion.

Whitney gets to the hospital at 7:45 a.m. and begins sprinting immediately. She finds she must make herself very small, very physically unobtrusive in order to stay out of the way of the rushing doctors and the patients being wheeled at a running pace into different operating rooms. It's times like this that her background as a performer, dancer, and choreographer comes in handy. Doulas are regularly seen in the OR holding area rubbing lower backs, offering hot packs, using the power of talking and distraction (otherwise known as "verbicane") before the clients are able to actually have their procedure, sometimes for hours until it begins.

Most second trimester abortions aren't performed in hospitals; often that level of care is unnecessary. Even in the second trimester, abortion is a very safe, low-risk procedure.

But even safe procedures become risky in the face of preexisting medical issues. City Hospital is a referral site in New York City, which means that they care for patients who are too medically high-risk to have procedures performed in a freestanding clinic such as Planned Parenthood. Most of the clients at City Hospital are not people who could have easily obtained abortions. Often they began the process by going to another clinic in the city and being told that the procedure would need to be performed in a hospital setting. The clients are generally dealing with medical issues like anemia, epilepsy, aortic stenosis, and a dizzying list of other possibilities that make most freestanding abortion clinics inaccessible. In addition, many of the clients have had C-sections with previous pregnancies, which can create issues with the forming placenta. As the placenta gets larger and blood flow to the uterus increases, the risks of the procedure multiply with the possibility of blood loss.

Procedures here are a two- to three-day process and begin in clinic during laminaria insertions, where thin rods made out of sterile seaweed are placed in the opening of the cervix. The entire abortion procedure, known as a dilation and evacuation (D and E), is done vaginally, but—as the doctors often assert—good cervical dilation is important in order for it to be safe. The doctors, counselors, and doulas all have to remember this while supporting people through laminaria insertions. The general consensus from clients is that it's really uncomfortable. We tell patients that it feels somewhere between period cramps and labor contractions, with the added discomfort of a speculum exam and the knowledge that they're feeling this peculiar cramping sensation because someone put an object inside their cervix.

At City Hospital patients are given a local anesthetic and ibuprofen for their laminaria insertions, which serve to take the edge off the discomfort. But every client handles the procedure differently. Some do not find it to be all that bad, and there are a lot of clinics in New York that are able to give people more or better anesthesia for the laminaria. New York City has particularly open Medicaid coverage for abortion, and several public hospitals in New York will fee-scale abortion procedures according to a patient's income. In other places in the country where Medicaid will not cover abortions, patients will often use inadequate anesthesia to lower the expense of their abortions. At City Hospital, resources are available but must be stretched to their maximum capacity. Therefore, the amount of anesthesia offered is, at best, sufficient to minimal.

Once the laminaria are placed, clients are discouraged from changing their minds because of the potential risks to the pregnancy. That the laminaria mark a point of no return is something that Whitney finds humbling and profound, especially given that City Hospital usually has a weeklong wait for abortions and what feels like a hundred bureaucratic hoops to jump through to get to the OR. While it might seem cruel that after a long wait the procedure itself takes several days, Whitney notes that the pace can often be appropriate for clients—even soothing. Whitney describes:

You have begun a process that can't be reversed. In that,

there is something poetic. I heard from women that because it is a two- or three-day process, it allows the mind,
body, and person to integrate what's happening a little
differently. There is something about those few days for
women who have been pregnant longer that seems almost
like a support in a way, like they are able to mellow into the
reality of the decision.

By the time OR day arrives, the doulas and the clients
have spent one or two days together and formed a deep connection. Whitney says, "When you know you are going to
be with someone for a more medically intense and longer
experience, for me I felt more of a commitment to the situation. To reassure somebody that I will see her tomorrow and
I will be there is much different than [a first trimester abortion experience], where we're together for the next two or
three hours." She notes that having an extra few days means
"much more time with them. On OR days there is no way
for clients to distract themselves, so you are there to be that,
to be present and to be a diversion. It was hard to leave some
of them. I couldn't believe we would probably never see each
other again."

In general, the practice of medicine speaks to an algo-
rithm—a standardized "to-do" list that serves as a guideline
for any given procedure—but it is also hinged on provider
preference and style. Doctors will often do surgeries and
procedures based on how they were taught and what feels
comfortable or familiar to them. Abortion procedures are no
different, but only a small percentage of doctors are taught

to do second trimester abortions, so training is inconsistent. There are many different details in administering second trimester terminations that can vary widely from provider to provider. Typically they are either done by using medication to induce labor (the same medication used for early medical abortion, but more of it) or by dilation and evacuation.

The D and E is surgically unique due to the fact that it is a "blind" procedure: there is no incision. The doctors use their sense of touch and sometimes ultrasound guidance to perform the procedure. In a lot of ways it's very elegant—the body takes care of itself, the uterus cramps down and goes back to its original size, and there is no scar to say that anyone was ever there.

Whitney and other doulas have found that even if it is just a matter of building rapport, clients are relieved to see familiar faces in the operating room amid the waves of blue scrubs and bouffant caps and what feels like dozens of people they've never seen before. The OR space can be overwhelming, kind of like a casino but with medical equipment. Walking into the OR is like walking into the middle of a conversation where everyone has some knowledge you don't. There is no budget at City Hospital to soften the aesthetics of the space. There are no bright windows, no warm-colored paint; it always looks gray.

City Hospital's abortion service is only one small piece of a large puzzle of services. Second trimester abortions are only done on Thursdays—days filled with a lot of running around, a lot of drama, and a lot of optimistic time management that always ends up leaving hospital staff disappointed. But while waiting for her client, Whitney wants to be discreet. Most hospital staff are familiar with the "weird" volunteer doulas, but because much of the nursing staff leans pro-life, everyone politely avoids the topic of abortion. Half of the people the doulas see in the OR admire the care the doulas offer; the other half are vaguely horrified by it. People get promoted to administrative roles every time the wind blows, and you never know who is looking for a reason to remove the doulas from the OR— so it's always best to blend in.

In the meantime, patients getting a wide variety of other surgeries moan in the holding area. Whitney glides over to the best place in the entire OR: a heated metal storage unit filled with deliciously warm blankets. The doulas call it "the blanket oven," and we are all grateful for it because it is one of the few tangible resources we can offer our clients to manage their pain. Whitney takes advantage of the heat in her paper-thin scrubs as she brings blankets over to a man who has been moaning. She walks past the medical students and doctors' research interns who have muttered sympathies about the man but did not approach him. He thanks her profusely, and they chat for a moment. Whitney goes back to her post while an anesthesiologist talks to him about his allergies. The medical students and research interns quietly begin to get blankets for patients who are uncomfortable, shuffling through niceties. It is Doula Training 101.

Whitney's client, Shelly, comes into the holding area. She is fifteen or sixteen years old. A cheerleader with an anxiety disorder, her eyes are wide and brimming with panic. Her parents are upstairs in the waiting room. The laminaria have caused her to have painful cramping that lasted throughout the night. The doctors weren't able to get as many rods in as they wanted to, so she has been given medication to jump-start the cervical softening. Shelly looks visibly relieved when Whitney walks over.

Whitney speaks to her in soft, loving tones and rubs her lower back. Shelly blinks away tears. "I'm so scared," she half-whispers. "What is it going to be like?"

Whitney thinks about the operating room itself and how to describe it. This is a common question, along with whether the client will wake up during the procedure, how it will all be different when it's over, and if she will feel like herself again. She tries to mitigate Shelly's fear. She describes the space, the gymnastics of scooting from the gurney to the operating table, and how Shelly will be asleep shortly after the anesthesia is given. Whitney says, "You might see a lot of equipment, but most of it will never be used." She does not say what she remembers of her own experience with anesthesia: *You might feel really out of your body and really sad for weeks and weeks.*

The client nods and curls into herself. She is curved, clenched—a seashell, wrapped in warm blankets.

"Will you come in with me?"

"I am going to be with you no matter what."

When it's time to go into the OR, Whitney grabs a surgical mask and walks swiftly to Shelly's right side, stepping out of the way of the anesthesiologists and the nurses who are busy making her as comfortable as possible. Whitney locks eyes with Shelly, hoping she will not fear the operating table that is covered in equipment and placed within the doctors' reach "just in case."

The doctors give Whitney space to do her work, keeping Shelly comfortable. She alternates between casual conversation—"What do you think you want to eat after the procedure?" "What's your favorite subject in school?"—and soothing reinforcement. Shelly is injected with the anesthesia while Whitney holds her right hand. Whitney understands keenly that the way someone goes to sleep is often similar to the way that she will wake up, so she focuses on keeping Shelly calm. In the background, music is playing. The doctors talk quietly about their upcoming vacations and the weather.

The doulas almost all say that they expect a certain reverence to fill the OR during an abortion, an air that is hushed, respectful, sometimes somber, and maybe even celebratory. Many of us came into the space and, instead, found ourselves offended by anything and everything that wasn't sweet, sensitive, and patient focused. Many of us also had the experience of our patients joining in on the very conversations we were bothered by, so we realized that we could be a little lighter too. We are often surprised when we see that for some people, especially the doctors and the nurses who do surgeries and abortions all day, every day, sometimes it is just a job. It is one of countless subtleties Whitney has figured out, along with where to stand (when you are new to an OR, you feel chronically in the way, because you are), how to manage her body language, when to step in and help, when to back off, the timing of the procedure, and the culture of the room.

As the anesthesia goes in, it burns a little. Shelly squeezes Whitney's hand tight before her grip loosens with sleep. Whitney lets go so that the procedure can begin, and it is this moment of letting go that is her most emotional experience. Everything gets moving, and the doctors get to business. They hold Shelly's head back and intubate her. The Reproductive Choices team gets ready to do the procedure. Whitney is not squeamish: in her role as a biomechanical healer, she has done cadaver dissections and by this point, she has seen many D and Es. Though they are an eyeful, they do not necessarily bother her. There is a lot less blood than she had first expected. But she does acknowledge that the procedure unavoidably resembles a birth. There is a big range of growth between fourteen weeks and the legal limit of twenty-four weeks; often City Hospital's clients are somewhere between eighteen and twenty-two weeks. It would be reductive to say that the procedure is gory—although it is. In our exposure to the OR, many doulas will attest that much of what you see or hear or smell accidentally, from any of the surgeries in any of the operating rooms, seems gory or violent. It can be hard to watch at times, but this is a crucial part of what the doulas do—it is not about our feelings or beliefs in that moment.

Whitney says that she did not have much of a connection to the physical procedure, but that in attending D and Es every week, "I kept thinking how different [my client's] life

94

was going to be afterward. [My goal was] just empowering that decision and her life afterward and how just fucking great that is for her to step in there and say, 'This is what I need to do even if I have to surrender and give you my body and my consciousness for an hour.'"

Whitney takes a quiet moment to survey the room before stepping out to check on the other clients in recovery, maybe even to rest while there is some precious downtime. She describes the OR as having three chapters:

> There's the prologue, the actual procedure, and the epilogue. The prologue is when she goes to sleep. The procedure is just this mass of material and skin and tissue, and the parts of this woman that she created and grew, and it's not there anymore and would have had potential. And all of the hormonal processes just stop. And then the epilogue, once the procedure is finished, is where I feel the most drawn. The patients are put to sleep, and when they wake up things are physically different. They are put into a recovery room with lots of other people who had everything *but* a termination done. Often even if [my clients] don't feel like crying or didn't want to give me a hug or anything [before the procedure], they generally did afterward. They were feeling relief or grief or fatigue or fear. I had such a hard time leaving. I felt like I could be there forever.

Whitney floats through the long hall of the operating room. She checks in on the client who came in before Shelly who is getting ready to leave, walking out into the crisp autumn weather with a look of hard-won relief. She gives the client a long hug before she heads back downstairs, and the client thanks her for being there. She decided with her partner to have the abortion, but he couldn't take off of work to be with her. She says to Whitney as she pulls her shoes on, "You made me feel safe."

Whitney doesn't feel like she did much, and she is grateful for these words. Sometimes it's hard to tell how your role is manifesting for your client. Whitney says, "You get to know them and have this incredibly intimate experience that no one else in their life is having with them. It's strange to be a doula in some ways—not the intimacy of the experience but that maybe a client would rather have a friend, or a partner, or a family member with her." Yet here Whitney is in this privileged position partially because—like most abortion services—City Hospital does not let patients bring their own support person to the procedure room. She has to fill the role of this support person without any knowledge of what the client might need. To do this she says, "I try to always approach every situation with as much humility as I can. I don't know what you're experiencing and it could change instantaneously. But there is power in that too. Whatever you are feeling, there is [the] possibility to shift it. With some of [the clients] we would end up joking and laughing at other things in their life or the situation itself."

She runs back downstairs. Shelly's procedure might be over by now, and Whitney is worried that coming out of the anesthesia might be distressing for her. She is right. Shelly is in the recovery room now in the throes of a panic attack, somewhere between awake and delirious and still half-asleep—a nightmarish combination. She is sobbing and screaming, asking for her parents. Whitney calls her name, and Shelly recognizes her voice. She leans into Whitney's open arms and cries into her shoulder.

A small group of nurses divides and conquers. One asks Whitney to try to get the patient to breathe deeply so that her heart rate goes down and her oxygen goes up; Shelly is starting to hyperventilate. Another tries to comfort the other patients on either side of the thin cloth curtains around Shelly, both of whom are also recently out of who-knows-what surgeries, and are disturbed by the commotion. Two other nurses loudly scold Shelly for having an abortion "so late" and telling her she "shouldn't have done it." Whitney whispers soothing things into her ear, hoping she doesn't hear the callous remarks. Finally, another nurse attempts to call the psychiatry service, which feels to Whitney like shooting a fly with a shotgun, especially when Shelly gets upset at the idea of seeing another new person. Shelly moans that she wants her mom and holds Whitney tighter. Whitney does her best to comfort her so that she will at least breathe but wishes she could do more. She asks one of the nurses to call the OR where the Reproductive Choices doctors are.

Attending physician Dr. A walks in with her characteristic stride. Dr. A can be succinctly described as "unfuckwithable." She is warm but imposing, unapologetically blunt in her speech, and fiercely protective of her service. Whitney tells her that Shelly is asking for her mother.

Dr. A asks loudly, "What's the problem?" She speaks to the nursing manager of the recovery room, and in ten minutes

Shelly's mother appears. Shelly is immediately calmer though still a bit shaken. Whitney checks the time—her shift ended twenty minutes ago, and she needs to get to work. There is another doula ready to take her place on the OR floor. But it's hard for Whitney to go. She strokes Shelly's hair and whispers goodbye, squeezing her mother's arm.

Sometimes Whitney leaves the hospital and doesn't know what to do with herself. She chronically wonders "how to complete those experiences and feel those experiences in real time and encapsulate them. What do you say? 'Bye, I love you?' You don't say that, yet you have this love for this person that you will probably never see again, and you never saw before that week. And you also have reverence for everyone involved, like *everyone* involved. The guys that come clean the room. Everyone."

Whitney has a bad habit of scheduling herself without a buffer, giving herself only enough time to get from one commitment to another. She pedals her bike across the city to her paid job, feeling something along the lines of "haunted" but better. Whitney feels now, as she has felt so many times before, that she needs to process the experience of the day but doesn't know how. She comes home and finds her clients are with her, the three or four people she cared for. She has "a love and vulnerability and tenderness now that doesn't have a place to go." She says, "I don't know what to do with that energy because it feels valuable. It is compassion and has a tone and a shape after these days."

She has learned that she has to give herself a little more

time to absorb or process what she experienced. Whitney says that, "I found it was in my subconscious pretty deeply. I would have dreams about the women and really be thinking about them for the day after. I would wonder, how are they today? Are they home yet? Did everything work out? How do they feel now that they aren't at the hospital?"

She remembers that on the day of her own abortion a patient walked out—just decided she wasn't going to do it. It struck Whitney, who was waiting patiently by the window in her medical gown and her hospital socks. She wondered what was going to happen with her.

During her pregnancy, which was short, Whitney says that she "didn't feel so pregnant." She thinks about that against the length of time that her second trimester clients have lived with the major shifts and changes pregnancy can bring physically, emotionally, and mentally. Sometimes her abortion comes back to her in waves, prompted by both the OR and other experiences. During the part of her abortion that most people find to be painful, toward the end when the procedure was about to be over, Whitney held Lauren's hand and softly repeated to herself, "It's okay . . . it's okay . . ."

It was the same thing she repeated when she was mugged several years back, which resulted in multiple reconstructive surgeries. "All the times, in all these other ways, I'm really hurt and I'm left in pieces, not being able to say, 'It's not okay.' I never felt like it was okay to say that. I know now it is. In that situation you're like, 'Well I want this over as quickly as possible.' There is no way to stop and ask, 'What has you upset right now? What exactly is going on?'"

Many of us come to this work because of an impulse toward compassion. For many of us, that also comes from a place of implicit or embedded trauma, maybe a desire to make right for other people what we have perceived as being so wrong for ourselves. Not all doulas come to the work because of trauma, but many caregivers of all stripes and of all genders find that the intimacy of bearing witness to these experiences can bring up a lot. Revelations come unprompted. If you are lucky, it is also a resolution.

For Whitney, doula care prompted her to look directly at her own history of trauma: sexual abuse, her mugging, her abortion. Without meaning to, she found that in bearing witness to others she held up a mirror to herself. She says:

> Anything someone goes through, she can survive and thrive afterward . . . No one I ever met [in the OR] felt like it was a nothing situation or a light situation. No patient I was ever with was like, "This is not a big deal." For those in second trimester it was a big deal on some level. And I was floored by the clients. I was humbled by them, thinking, "You are so much stronger than I could ever imagine being. I am so honored to be in this space with you. I'm learning so much." It's not about you [when you're] a doula or what you are doing, but . . . it's an exchange of energy and information and experience. I just hope we make it a day where they also have an experience of kindness and surrender.

Whitney goes home full of compassion and gratitude, feeling dropped straight down into the "realness" of it. She thinks about how her life has changed because of this work.

She tries to understand the reasons why it is so important to her and such a part of her, but she can only see the tenuousness of life and an urge—almost primal—to keep going. She unlocks her door and walks in, thinking of everyone who becomes shaped and changed by this work: the doulas, the doctors, the clients.

"Everyone on every side of it. It's the women, it's their children, it's the partners. It's profound. And we don't even really know. You just step in, you don't even know what effects this might have. I'm going to try to do my best to create positive waves and forgive when I don't. There's a kind of poetry in my life and in everyone's. There's so much grace."

All the Way
Lauren and Jonna

Jonna has spent this entire pregnancy running in circles. She has just turned thirty-nine and is getting ready to send her daughter—her one and only baby—to college. Last year Jonna's mother passed away, and she lost the key support person in life. She is still in a haze of mourning, emotionally limping after the loss. She has recently been laid off from her nonprofit job, where she had been a loyal worker even when things weren't going well for the organization. Her relationship with her partner vacillates between crappy and "okay enough." He has placed his disapproval for Jonna's decision at her feet and otherwise remains absent throughout the process.

The decision to have an abortion or not is salt in the wound of Jonna's tumultuous year. Never having had to make this choice before, she is conflicted from the start. She asks herself, *Why me? Why now?* Nearly forty years old, with a child almost out of the house, and *now* she has an unintended pregnancy? What shit luck.

Jonna was not expecting to be a single mother for her first daughter, and yet—things happen; she knows that. She tells people that she was strong, and is strong, because she has no other choice. Now she's confronting the possibility of being a single mother all over again. She says "possibility" not because she doesn't have faith in her partner—there is love between them—but because the pregnancy brings up cracks in their foundation that maybe otherwise wouldn't have been a problem. The "possibility" of being a single mother is apparent to Jonna simply because she knows that there can always be that possibility.

When she moves forward with the decision to have the abortion, the choice remains halfhearted—cloaked in ambivalence. She really doesn't know what's worse: having a baby or doing something to stop that from happening. She feels sick and nauseous, possibly from the pregnancy itself or from the anxiety that makes its home in the pit of her stomach. She misses her mother. She does not tell anyone about the pregnancy. She does not want that judgment in her most vulnerable moment.

When she finally decides to have an abortion, she goes to Planned Parenthood and receives some bad news: they can't do her procedure. Fibroid cysts have grown all over her uterus, making the procedure unsafe to perform at a freestanding clinic.

She is handed City Hospital's number, and her heart drops. *Is this a sign?*

Jonna tries to ask what will happen if she goes full term with the pregnancy. The responses are vague, unfulfilling, anxiety provoking: "We just don't know." She hears about a friend of a friend who had a stillbirth in her ninth month of pregnancy, ostensibly because of bad fibroids. Jonna feels her chest tighten at the idea of going through months of wondering, anticipating bad news. Everything feels like the wrong decision.

She takes some time to think before calling City Hospital and drags her feet a little before she commits. When she finally calls, she is invited to be an agent of her own care in a web of bureaucracy. By now she has entered her second trimester, and her fibroids have continued to grow with the blood flow to her uterus. Some of them are huge and uncomfortable. At a certain point she is warned, the fibroids may run out of space in her body or will exhaust their blood supply. They will then begin to die, causing excruciating pain in the last half of her pregnancy. Given the amount, size, and placement of the fibroids, no one can offer much information about whether they will negatively impact the fetus. No one will know that answer until, most likely, she is past the legal limit of abortion.

Jonna sees images in her head of the baby being crushed by her own body. A nightmare.

By the time Jonna is in City Hospital's waiting room she has been dealing with this decision for over a month. I meet her when Melissa, my mentor and senior counselor in the clinic, calls her into our office. Today I am wearing my "counselor" and not my "doula" hat. After several years I know the difference between the two well, even if they look the same at times. I jokingly call Melissa my "work wife" when we realize that we see each other more than anyone else in our lives. It's a form of life partnership where we know we will always be bonded because no one outside of this office will really understand what it's like to do our job—or at least not in this way in which our lives work in tandem. Melissa and I often do something along the lines of cocounseling, the two of us working with the patients at once. Mostly this happens while we are coordinating appointments within the mayhem of City Hospital; we are one small piece of a gargantuan system. Our shared office is roughly the size of a postage stamp. We try to make it homey, even though it's supposed to look very "clinical" according to hospital standards. We gently place funny posters amid the birth control and STD information, colorful Post-it notes cheering for one another on our desks. We make furniture out of the giant boxes of health department NYC-brand condoms that they send to us way too often.

Before Jonna comes in, we see a copy of her medical chart. Our eyes zero in on the ultrasound report that shows a blurry gray image of a uterus knotted with over a dozen large fibroids. We've seen patients with fibroids like this before. We've discussed at many different points how we rarely feel surprised anymore at our high-risk mess of an institution, where all problems are unique and yet rarely singular. We try to use our jaded affect to our advantage: "How will we do it this time?" We are well practiced, well versed. This is our normal.

We scramble to rearrange our packed surgical schedule,

and find a way to squeeze Jonna into our once-a-week operating room patient waiting list. We sprint to figure out the "hows" and "whens" and "wheres" of her appointments. It is one of many moments when I have to resist defining a patient by her medical history before I meet her in person. In order to properly advocate for her in the giant monolith that is City Hospital, Melissa and I make calls and repeat over and over again the description of Jonna's fibroids. I wonder what image people have of her—at this point, for all we know of Jonna, she might as well be a uterus with legs. Melissa and I—realizing this—sigh and look over at one another like the old married couple we've become.

Jonna comes in statuesque, regal, even in her casual jeans and T-shirt. She is friendly but distracted. Between waiting for all of her appointments and realizing that her options are limited and her procedure will require extra care and finesse, time has melted away. This is the case for many of City Hospital's patients; the service is small but intense, and very few people have medical needs that are straightforward. Even though City Hospital is always working at its maximum capacity, resources are few. We do the best we can, but it feels like it will never be enough. It won't be—a few people can't act as the Band-Aids for the massive issues that come with healthcare.

Melissa starts the conversation with Jonna while I get everything ready for the next patient, trying to keep the day under control by staying on top of the well-oiled machine of the clinic. We are notified that yet another patient—a third patient—is ready to be seen, and a fourth is yelling and frustrated in the waiting room. It is a typical day, and in many ways not memorable. Jonna is one of countless patients who unexpectedly finds herself labeled "medically complicated" during her pregnancy, even though she has been healthy all her life. She is told to scramble to a list of appointments, all given to her in a tone of insistence typically reserved for patients we worry won't appreciate how important the details are. In the end, it's a game of "hurry up and wait."

With one ear, I follow the urgent conversation. "You *must* come to this appointment." "You *can't* miss this." "*Please* communicate with us." "You *have to* stay for another ultrasound today—no, another one, a better one," and so on. Jonna nods. She is frustrated, but at least she is gracious. I wish we could make it easier for her. But that road leads to madness; we can't lubricate the system more than we already do. There are no heroes in bureaucracy.

I was hired by City Hospital several months after we launched the Doula Project in 2008. On the surface it seemed like an ideal match, since I had taken on the role of a sexual health counselor informally for years. I had the dubious honor of being one of the earlier bloomers to hit sexual awakening in my mostly Catholic and, by extension, slut-shaming high school. Afraid to tell anyone that I was doing "it" and abjectly horrified of becoming pregnant after one scare, I learned to clandestinely take the bus to Planned Parenthood a few towns over to get birth control pills. There, I would hoard information packets every time I went. I thought they would be useful. I would bury my face in my new reading material—"Should YOU get a pap smear?"—and walk past the antiabortion protesters with their graphic signs to get back on the bus. Through the window, a woman with fluffy bangs who always wore the same brown plaid skirt and held the same sign with a picture of a fetus in a bucket, would mouth, "They don't care about you." I would shrug in response.

When I started hearing whispers of other people losing their virginities a year or so later, I decided to try to save them the trouble of collecting information at Planned Parenthood. I publicly outed myself as "knowing too much" when—during a health class—I corrected a speaker. People had mostly gotten past the point of being overly mean to one another about it; now, they needed the information too. I became the go-to person for friends and friends of friends who needed answers. I learned to put on a good "counselor" face—the kind that is soft, with eyebrows slightly knit together, a hint of a warm smile, sweet and empathetic eyes, an occasional affirmative nod—as I fielded question after question: "Yes, you can get pregnant your first time." "No, condoms are not 100 percent effective." "Oral gonorrhea can actually happen; there's an outbreak in town now." "No, you can't get pregnant from swallowing." "Yes, anal counts."

Years later, at the time we started the Doula Project, I was mostly freelancing as a doula and a writer and failing at both. The instability of "freelance" life was not a good fit. I found out really fast that I was bad at asking people for money, *especially* for doula work. And, coming from a family background where money struggles were pressing for much of my life, I was at an impasse where I wouldn't have much of a safety net if I failed. Trips to pawnshops were frequent. With my jaw set and my face stony, as if I weren't desperate, I offered up some of the few unsentimental nice things I had with the goal of getting twenty dollars in a pinch. My family and my partner at the time were encouraging and helped as much as they could, but my independence was in question. I felt like I was bad at being an adult, that my college scholarship had gone to waste because I chose to do an interdisciplinary humanities degree, which stared back at me blankly during more than a few dark times that year.

To make ends meet, I worked as a creative-writing teacher in public middle schools and worked in medical education as a "standardized patient" and a gynecological teaching associate (GTA). Part of this involved acting; I was given a script with a list of symptoms and a brief character summary. Medical students were then tested on their social skills based on how well they interacted with my character, which—because I have looked the same since age fifteen—was usually a sexually active teenager with an ectopic pregnancy. (As a sidenote, I found that teaching social skills to adolescents was remarkably the same as teaching them to medical students.) Being a GTA was a little more intensive. I would teach medical students how to do comprehensive, patient-centered gynecological exams using my own body as a tool. My colleague Laura Duncan, also a GTA, affectionately calls it being a "speculum jockey." It was equal parts incredible, empowering, and hilarious; my knowledge of vaginas became encyclopedic.

But these small projects weren't enough. When I was offered the job at City Hospital, I was so broke that the hospital vending machines rejected my change for being too small. Health insurance and a regular paycheck sounded *real* good.

The Doula Project became my rock and my coping mechanism at a time when everything felt in flux for me. During those first few months, being at the clinic gave me a high—like I had an abundance of love to give to almost anyone who needed it. It was new and refreshing to be here after feeling irate for so long at the levels of systemic injustice that informed my reasons for stepping into doula work in the first place.

I come to this work from the perspective of embodiment and trauma, my own history of embodied trauma—a sexual assault at a young age—notwithstanding. It has never been something I've found easy naming outright, nor sharing. But whether or not I wanted to admit it (or want to admit it, even now), there was something I hoped to make better for others that I felt I was failing at making better for myself, or at the very least, that I knew had potential to be so haunting, and so damaging, without love and support from community. How can you find your way home, back to yourself, when you feel shattered? Or say out loud, "I need to be held with both hands, and I'm not sure I can do it alone?" Because for me, asking for help is the peak moment of vulnerability. Receiving love and care when it's offered is easier.

So if I couldn't find it in myself (find what? Words? Strength? I still don't know) to ask for what I needed, I could at least offer first, from an intuitive place. I taught speculum exams to medical students because it seemed like a tangible, useful solution to real problems—teaching doctors how to be compassionate in the face of the physical and emotional vulnerability of their patients—while also giving me space to reclaim something in myself. I became a birth doula, did all this "stuff" because trauma inflicted on the body takes on a living, breathing reality. It takes on a separate life inside you, a part of you, but fragmenting. It's something that has been theorized and talked about at length, and of course, it feels different for everyone. A lot of people will agree that it's insidious: it creeps in and darkens the edges of your perspective when you least expect it.

I started working in reproductive justice to fight back against a system that covers everything like Saran Wrap, a thin but almost unbreakable film. I got involved in medicine for these reasons, which I would only be able to articulate later. In the beginning it was, "OMG I want to do this because OMG awesome and OMG radical." It is easy to allow the desire to seek justice for others eclipse our responsibility to look at ourselves because—for many of us—that's what hurts without respite, without the clarity of logical answers, unclouded by emotions or distress. That's what we know will take a lifetime to fix.

Being hired at City Hospital was good for me as a person and was a good strategic move for the Doula Project. It meant that our open-ended "partnership" with City Hospital could become solidified because someone on the inside could advocate for it. It also meant that in the first year and a half of the program when Mary and I were handling most of our clients, I truly felt the weight of working two full-time direct-care jobs. I felt like my life was now contextualized by stories that weren't mine. I knew that I loved what I was doing and that I loved my clients even though I didn't really know them and wouldn't see most of them again.

The hospital became my home away from home; it felt like I was always there but not necessarily in a bad way. I often went to sleep at night exhausted, sometimes covered in bodily fluids that weren't mine, with my clients' voices in my ear. On good nights the voices would say "thank you" and repeat the sweet words spoken throughout the day. It wasn't the only reason I was there, but let's face it: you need something like that, something positive that comes back to you. It solidified for me how wonderful my patients were and confirmed that they made all of the hard parts of this job worth it. And it made me feel okay to ask for help when I needed it, to let my guard down, and to know that most people are very kind—that most of our clients want to take care of us just as we want to take care of them.

Later, when Jonna comes to check in, she tells me that she recognizes me. We have a mutual friend. The line of professionalism gets a little blurry, but so does the hierarchy that comes from a pseudo-therapeutic relationship. We become very human to one another, all at once.

Jonna, Melissa, and I all get in touch a minimum of once a day for about a week. Our banter is friendly, familiar.

An ultrasound with a good machine, a trained sonographer, and a specialist in high-risk pregnancy care show that one of Jonna's fibroids is resting like a boulder on her cervix, distorting its shape and position. Jonna hears this, but it doesn't mean much until the providers speak in English instead of medicalese: "This will not be easy."

Normally the abortion process begins by placing the laminaria dilators through the opening, or "os," of the cervix. Unfortunately, this process may not be possible for Jonna if the doctors are unable to see the opening of the cervix or if the fibroid has made the cervix itself longer than the dilators.

A short list of unappealing options unfurls before Jonna. Dizzying medical terms take on new life as they are rapidly demystified with every new line on the consent form: hysterectomy, hysterotomy, labor induction, procedures that require "ultrasound guidance" and an ominous-sounding needle. Jonna's brow furrows though she otherwise appears composed. Her cigarette breaks become long, frequent, and necessary—like breaths of air. They are one of the few signs that she is struggling with this decision.

I review the procedure options with her by rote. I am distracted as I speak because of how much it all just sucks. We talk about her options before the doctors arrive and I toe the line of my multiple roles: doula, counselor, and frequent mouthpiece for the doctors. I give her the lowdown on the process, trying to be frank yet compassionate while negotiating which boundaries of what professional role I need to adhere to.

Jonna is not someone who wants or needs sugarcoating. She has the option to attempt the procedure in the "normal" way, using the dilator rods before the surgical dilation and evacuation. She can choose to induce labor using medications, but that involves going to the labor floor with all of the birth accoutrements that every other laboring person gets, including a crew of pro-life labor and delivery nurses who are blunt in their disdain for anything abortion related. She can do a hysterotomy: an early C-section that will need a vertical incision that could cause more damage to her uterus in the long run. It is a complicated, uncomfortable procedure with a long recovery period. Or—since she feels she doesn't want another baby—she can, in the name of efficiency, do a "gravid hysterectomy" and remove the fibroids and the fetus along with her uterus.

If a "regular" abortion procedure can't be done, the doctors, bluntly practical as they are, feel that the gravid hysterectomy is best. They are cavalier about it, though not unkind. They live in a world where surgery is normal, a means to an end. They're detached from the fear or mourning of losing an organ. Even so, it is ironic that because of the fibroids the hysterectomy offers the least amount of physical risk.

Jonna reviews her options. Though she delivered her daughter by C-section she balks at the idea of doing it again. "For what?" she asks. It is too much pain and too much surgery. She gives that option a firm no. And she absolutely doesn't want a hysterectomy.

When she chooses labor induction, even I cringe. More than half of the births I've attended as a doula have been labor inductions. It has become an accidental specialty of mine, starting from when the Doula Project came to City Hospital and came across clients who would have been completely alone during their stillbirths were it not for a doula. My connection with these clients has always been especially strong.

I worry about Jonna's decision to do a labor induction, because it is a birth. She would have to be involved and awake throughout the entire process. Labor inductions aren't easy for anyone, but more often than not the people who choose them are doing so because of fetal anomalies: genetic or congenital issues that often lead to a grim outcome if the pregnancy is brought to term. The clients who opt for labor induction typically want time to see and hold the baby; they want time to say goodbye.

Some clients are under the impression that labor induction would be more "natural" or easier or safer than the surgical abortion. Many think of their own birth experiences with other children, and they feel more comfortable doing that than they do dealing with the drama of having a surgical abortion. It's a rude awakening when they realize that a labor induction is not very "natural" at all. Clients are given medications to start the labor and IVs with fluids. They are strapped to monitors—they can't move, they can't eat, and their contractions are often so bad that they choose an epidural. According to physician David Grimes, the uterus is not evolved to deliver a pregnancy during the second trimester. Miscarriages usually happen in the first trimester, and babies are delivered in the third, at the end of the pregnancy. Labor inductions in the second trimester can be as long and arduous as any full-term birth but with more medications. In other words—not a natural birth process.

My mind races through the other inductions I have

attended. Several of my clients, like Jonna, had never experienced a vaginal delivery. Those clients tended to have a harder time, if only because of the newness of the physical feeling and the newness of the "birth" experience overall. Jonna had never even felt labor contractions. When she had her daughter, she was brought straight in for a C-section. I try to think of ways to communicate some of the more brutal facts, like how she might hear newborn babies crying if the floor gets busy, without scaring her.

"Jonna, are you sure this feels like the best option for you?" As if I would know better. But on the tip of my tongue is the exact phrase that the doctors have been repeating in favor of the gravid hysterectomy: *You don't want more kids!*

I don't say that. "It's just that . . . It's not going to be easy. You'll be on the same floor as people who are delivering live babies. And it's a pretty dramatic, uncomfortable process. I just want you to be prepared . . ."

"Lauren, it's *my* uterus. And I'm not going to have a C-section. I'm not going to go through all of that for nothing, just to go home empty-handed."

When I ask her who will be with her during the labor induction, which I tell her could take anywhere from twelve to thirty-six hours, she shrugs. "I might have a friend come visit for a while," she says.

Her partner, in his tacit disapproval, will not be coming. "This is your decision," he said. And then his hands came off the issue. I have seen this before too. There have been many times when doulas get called because our clients' friends or family aren't actually able to stay, sometimes because they don't want to. My least favorite version of this story is when a client's family or friends will convince her to do a labor induction instead of an abortion procedure and then they all leave. It's something that I honestly couldn't imagine doing alone. And yes, it happens, and no, people are not breakable, but no one should have to do it alone if they have the option not to.

Jonna is trying to be strong and resolute through all of this. Later when I compliment her strength, she will sigh deeply and say with resignation, "Lauren, I am strong because I don't have another choice. I have to be."

But in this moment I offer Jonna the option of a doula and I speak broadly. She perks up and agrees that it sounds like a good idea. I'm surprised; vulnerability doesn't seem to come naturally to Jonna. But she is glad to have someone there. We are both glad when we realize that "someone" will be me.

We hug and finalize plans. Jonna is to come back later in the evening, and we agree that I will come meet her in the morning unless she calls and wants me to come earlier. For me it is a privilege to know in advance when I'm going to come back to the hospital. I savor the rest of the night, appreciating the basic luxuries of eating a nice dinner at a table and sleeping in a bed instead of curled over in my own lap in a delivery room.

I pull my blanket tightly around me and mentally prepare. As if in homage, I think of the faces of my previous stillbirth clients. I think of their names; I think carefully—in as much detail as I can—about their birth experiences. I fall into a hazy sleep that is barely restful; I wake up and feel like I've been running.

The morning stings with cold even though it's spring. I get to the hospital early, wearing my Keds and oversized blue scrubs, feeling like a small child in a doctor costume on Halloween. I find out that Jonna arrived several hours later than she was expected—this has been a running theme—and had to wait for hours before she was finally given a room. The residents scolded her for her lateness and then were surprised when she became ornery.

I walk to her room. I pass the nurses' station and wave. Some wave back; others roll their eyes. "Oh, it's *you*," one says. This is the same nurse who yelled at me the year before, asking why a patient who was "killing her baby" should have a doula while also complaining about how annoying doulas are. Grumblings about abortion being murder abound. A few turn it into friendly chatting and have come to like me as a person even if they believe I am an abortion-monger.

Jonna is alone, lying in bed with the TV on. She is annoyed, tired, and hungry but limited to hospital Jell-O and clear liquids. She points to a chair so I can sit.

The chair is a telltale sign that the nurses were expecting me. Most rooms have recliners so that the guests and partners of laboring patients can sit comfortably, maybe even sleep if they want. But as the nurses remind me, I am not a guest. I work here. "We save the good chairs for people who need them." The chair in here is the kind with a backrest that stops right before your shoulder blades. Its metal armrests form a halfhearted loop and reappear as a part of said backrest. It all leaves you sitting at some weird forward-leaning angle with a rod in your back.

I try to get comfy. Jonna dozes in and out.

As the day progresses, I respond to work emails, pick up trashy magazines for us to read, and clandestinely swallow LUNA bars in the hallway. The medication is moving through her system, but Jonna doesn't feel any major contractions yet. We are both anxious about that. The doctors have said that the cervical softener might not help melt that one huge cervical fibroid away. There is nothing to do but wait. We talk about everything and nothing; our conversations are easy, comfortable.

At one point, Jonna's brother stops in to see her. Jonna mentions to him that she met me after I gave a birth control talk at her former nonprofit job. She looks wryly at me. "I can't remember if it was a good talk because I didn't really listen to it." She looks at her brother. "I should have listened."

The induction starts to pick up speed at some point in the evening, Jonna's contractions intensifying. I keep an ear on "where" she feels the pain, trying to determine the answer to everyone's favorite question: "How much longer?" Of course, I wouldn't be able to tell her that, but I follow the arc of the labor from general cramping to back pain to vaginal pressure. Jonna is able to talk to me through her contractions. I rub her back and her legs, attempting to distract her during the peak of her discomfort. We both know we have a long way to go.

Eventually the contractions become predictably unbearable. I had expected Jonna to get an epidural like most clients who have labor inductions. In fact, it doesn't even cross my mind that she won't. I had seen enough disasters to feel very humble toward the epidural (which I describe to my clients unsentimentally as "having a giant needle in your spinal column"), but stillbirth inductions are brutal. The contractions are long, hard, and painful, and they come rapidly. Clients are mostly stuck in bed, unable to move. There really isn't much aside from the epidural that will relieve the pain of it.

Yesterday when Jonna and I spoke about the nuts and bolts of labor inductions, I mentioned that morphine would be an option for pain relief but that it wasn't very effective against contractions and would make her very nauseous. We agreed that it sounded terrible.

So I am shocked when Jonna asks for morphine instead of an epidural. "But . . . why?" I ask as I rub her lower back with a warm washcloth. *Jonna is full of surprises,* I think.

"This is manageable. This is like my period. I've heard too many crappy things about the epidural. I don't want it."

Being a doula means that you follow your client's lead even if you're not sure that's what you would do if you were in the same situation. Being a doula means it's not about you. Jonna is clearly comfortable taking the initiative in her own care. She gets her IV of morphine and is able to take the world's most delicious naps for about thirty seconds at a time before the contractions wake her. She vomits at the peak of her contractions. To me this looks hellish. To Jonna it is tolerable.

She is eventually able to doze off for a solid stretch of sleep. Every time she stirs, I bolt awake to rub her back, get her a warm compress, or replenish her fluids. This may seem overly vigilant, but it isn't. This is what doulas are trained to do and how most of us operate. Her contractions get steadily worse and she moans and breathes through them. I try using pressure points, peppermint oil, and massage. It feels both futile and "better than nothing." Finally, with one sleepy eye open, Jonna says, "Lauren, stop. Go to bed. You're not going to take this away."

That's a phrase I always find hard as a doula, though I've heard it many times before. I think many doulas badly want to take their clients' pain away. I especially wish I could during the stillbirths.

Our eyes lock, both bleary—mine, because I am exhausted; Jonna's because she is both exhausted and high as a kite from the morphine. She tells me firmly, "Go sit down. Put your feet on my bed. That's it . . . I'll let you know when I need you."

I fall asleep curled in on myself while Jonna squeezes my foot.

At around five in the morning, Jonna wakes me up because her water has broken. Often during these inductions everything happens at once: the water breaks and the fetus is delivered all in a matter of minutes.

I pop up and grab the doctors. There is no dramatic

pushing, only a lot of downward pressure. And then it's over, just like that.

At other stillbirths I have grown used to the choreography. Often the deliveries happen before any doctors can get into the room, which is generally not dangerous, even if it is jarring. I view my job as being to normalize everything as much as possible, keeping calm even when it feels like my heart is in my throat.

I will never forget the face of one would-be father who looked away and winced once the still, silent baby was delivered. Since then, I have always made it my business to pull a blanket over my clients' laps so that they don't have to see anything they don't want to see. I help wrap and swaddle the baby. I make the footprints. I learn baby names. I hear about plans that won't come to fruition, the new nursery that will get dismantled, and the toys, clothes, and bottles that will go back in their boxes. Many times I will weep with my clients.

Your job as a doula in these moments of anticipated crisis is to be calm, clear, and patient. To help create a safe space when the world is excruciating. It all changes you. You feel marked by every tear that falls on your shoulder, every little body in every little blanket. You go home and find that you are in mourning—maybe to some extent over the baby, but mostly for the loss your clients feel, the gap in their lives that they weren't expecting, the identity as a parent that they wanted but will not have at this time. You become grateful for everything you have and feel strength enough for only a happy life. You join people in their loss as much as they want you to. Sometimes they want you to be in as far as you can go.

Jonna's situation is somewhat different. Her decision-making process is complicated, but she does not see the baby as something that she knew she wanted. She doesn't want to hold the baby because she feels guilty. She says that this decision, being on the labor floor for an induction among other laboring mothers, is a "mindfuck." She feels it may have been masochistic. She doesn't like hearing about her own strength when she feels like she was only doing what was necessary.

After the delivery, when she is finally able to eat solids, we share a pastry. She says she is ready to leave this nightmare behind. She's ready to move on, if she can.

Healing for Jonna is complicated in all senses of the word. She must return to the hospital many times because the fibroids have caused extra bleeding that won't go away. In one of her many follow-up visits, she says she wants to be a doula; she wants to give something back. A year after her induction, Jonna joins the Doula Project. I'm excited because I know she'll be good at it, but I also only want her to do it if she is ready. She drags her feet for a while but is eventually able to doula at Planned Parenthood, far from City Hospital, where she hopes to process the experiences differently.

On her first day she meets a client who is unable to have her procedure in the clinic because she has fibroids on her uterus. Jonna remembers that caring for this client felt effortless because she could completely relate.

Twice a month for more than a year, she attended abortions at Planned Parenthood. She recalls that clients thanked her for all she did and hug her. It felt important because she understood the stakes of what she was doing. "I started doing this before I thought I really could," Jonna says to me now. "I did it for you because what you gave me by being there with me, when no one else was, was huge and important." She pauses. "But then I realized I needed this for me. And I haven't done it in a long time because I don't have time with my new job right now, but I know that I need this for me. It's for the clients, but it's also for me."

How to Pack a (Full-Spectrum) Doula Bag . . . And Unpack Assumptions

A mini chapter about some best practices we learned outside of our birth doula training, after years of working in direct care and utilizing the reproductive justice model. This chapter is specifically geared toward anyone who wants to become a full-spectrum doula.

Being a Great Activist Doesn't Make You a Great Doula

Having a strong social justice background is important for understanding the macro-level systems that may shape the experiences of our clients. The two of us began in the reproductive justice movement with backgrounds that were mostly steeped in advocacy, education, and organizing—not direct practice. But the learning curve to becoming a good doula is a sharp one. Part of doula work— especially in the way we define it—is attempting to change systems by working *within* them. It means that we have to push back against the injustices we see in our clinical spaces by being lovers, not fighters. It also means that change can be frustratingly slow, as you are now operating at the micro-level. The best doula work is able to bridge activism with individual care by helping pregnant people have empowered healthcare experiences and helping ensure that those experiences are voiced to society at large.

Be Aware of Your Own Power and Privilege

This is where the social justice background comes in. There is little education on anti-oppressive frameworks in the traditional birth-doula training course. To do this work, you have to be aware of your own power and privilege in the world, especially when you are dealing with systems like the very hospital or clinic where you are *volunteering.* The patient population at our clinic sites is extremely diverse. Many of our doulas haven't had half of the life experiences our patients have had, even when these patients are younger than us. It's not enough to expect that everyone will see the sincerity of your good intentions and trust you enough to open up to you. You learn fast to approach everyone with humility.

Nafeesa Dawoodbhoy of the SPIRAL Collective in Minneapolis, Minnesota, remembers, "I was surprised by how many of the more 'difficult scenarios' for abortion emotional support we went over in the training became relevant almost immediately on the job. I had initially thought, 'Oh, these scenarios are the extreme, most people won't be going through such serious emotions,' but as it turned out, the complexities of abortion for those who choose it became clear very soon. As an abortion doula, I had to confront people's issues with their faith, their spouses, their abusive relationships, domestic violence, and coercive reproduction all within the first month of the job."

Reproductive Healthcare Is Not "Empowering"

That's a bold statement, we know. But coming from a "re-productive rights" background, we went into the work with the hope that we would help people feel "empowered" in their decisions—no matter what they were. We soon learned that it's hard to feel empowered when you are dealing with any sort of intense physical process. For many people it can be a very fragmenting experience for the mind, body, and soul. Not to mention the imbalanced power dynamic that is often inherent between provider and patient. While it is our goal to reduce fear around birth and other reproductive processes, we can never predict where that fear is directed— unless we ask and listen. For many clients the key to feeling empowered, even in the face of bodily fear, is holding the knowledge that someone is really hearing you—even if they can't take away the anxiety. Poonam Dreyfus-Pai, who was a volunteer and member of the Leadership Circle of the Dou-la Project from 2009 to 2011 and codirector of the Bay Area Doula Project from 2012 to 2014, remembers:

> I'm funny because I knew—both for my abortion and birth trainings—that there was so much I still didn't know. I was super nervous right after training because I felt like I was supposed to know much more than I actually felt I did. It wasn't until my first shifts, when I could put the skills into action, that I could properly assess what I knew and where the gaps in my knowledge and practice were. Because I trained as an abortion doula first, I thought I was fully prepared for the kind of advocacy that doula-ing requires. As it turned out, it took a while to realize that

advocacy on behalf of a client requires, more than information and training, a listening ear. I had to learn to dial back the talking and offering of options. I actually didn't have to know everything; I just had to offer respectful, curious, empathetic listening so that people could allow their own wants, needs, and feelings to surface.

You Will Not Take Your Patient's Pain Away

This is a bitter, bitter pill to swallow. We all have our own reasons for becoming doulas, but most will say it is because they feel compelled to care for people during times of transition. Trying to be your clients' sword and shield to protect them from all badness will only lead you to realize the harsh limitations of what you can really do for them.

Learn to Be Comfortable with Being Uncomfortable

The constant position of a doula is to be a guest in someone else's house. This can be challenging, especially when you're first starting out. It's important to remember that sometimes saying that you're there to offer "compassionate patient care" can imply to clinic, hospital, or birthing center staff that they aren't doing that already. In addition, a lot of medical systems are overworked and a lot of staff members are exhausted. Sometimes doulas are greeted with skepticism in hospitals and clinics. It can be common to encounter brusque or curt attitudes. Sometimes you will feel like you have no idea where to stand or what you should be doing. You might always feel like you are "in the way." It's a skill to figure out where to be at any given time. Sometimes hospital or clinic policies might not make sense to people who are new or who don't have much experience working in medical facilities.

Dawoodbhoy thinks about the time she learned this lesson. "I crossed a line by accompanying a client out of the clinic [before she could actually leave] to get to her ride." Many of the issues that cause problems in clinics and hospitals are unintuitive unless you're there all day, every day. She points out, "Adhering to the rules that clinics impose, and balancing that with wanting to provide empathetic care, gives rise to a lot of gray areas. This is possibly the hardest thing to navigate as a doula."

Mirror the Language of Your Client

Within the first two weeks of being in the clinic, we learned that the word "abortion" was irrelevant to many of the people there, either because they were having abortion-like procedures to resolve miscarriages or because that word just didn't jive with them. Doulas also find that using words like "fetus" or "baby" can change how you are able to understand your client's relationship to her procedure.

Doula work and activism alike often target language as playing an important role in encouraging a shift toward inclusivity in culture. Part of our work is to consider the way that conversations around reproductive decisions on the individual level can impact public policy. The best way we have found to be sensitive to and inclusive of all of our clients and their experiences of their bodies is to repeat and reflect back to them whatever language they use.

Alternate the Tools of "Holding Space" and "the Gift of Gab"

We didn't appreciate when we were starting out just how much *waiting* there would be. We wait with patients in waiting rooms for clinic appointments and for their procedures. We wait with patients in recovery. We wait with patients to give birth after they've been given epidurals. Having a good talking rapport can be incredibly helpful during long stretches of time when you're hanging out with your client. It's a great way to give of yourself, to show that you're warm, and to begin to build trust. If you tend to be shy, keep a mental list of conversation topics ready (our favorites have to do with astrology and food). Dreyfus-Pai says:

> On the fly, I had to learn how to come up with great small talk! When I lived in New York, it was always easy to start with transportation—traffic, subway messes, etc. When I moved to California, I was doula-ing in a more rural place, so I learned a lot about farms in the area. One of the best things about making conversation was how willing and excited people were to talk about their kids—it was so easy to keep conversation interesting when you were asking about school, sports, Halloween costumes, Christmas presents. And I think it surprised people that I would ask, or would want to talk about their kids, while they were preparing for an abortion—in the beginning, I wasn't sure how to do it, or whether I would be awkward about it, but it actually came so naturally. The women I worked with *loved* their children, and it was so obvious that their deci-

sion to have an abortion was tied up with caring for the kids they already had. If that doesn't give you a full picture of people's reproductive lives—and the complexities they can hold—I don't know what does.

That aside, not everyone will feel like talking, and you don't want to push if you're getting signals that she's not into it. If your client seems detached or in her own head and doesn't want to be distracted, leave space for her to decline conversation. If she does, don't take it personally. See our earlier point about learning to be comfortable with being uncomfortable.

Learn Nonverbal Communication

Many of our clients are not native English speakers. Often they're not native Spanish or French speakers either. We might not even have a point of reference in a shared alphabet. Beyond language barriers, we also are confronted with cultural barriers. It is our job to figure out how to connect with our clients in spite of these challenges. Follow client cues and pay attention to body language. Often, clients appreciate kind words, even if they don't entirely understand what you're saying. Mime how to breathe deeply. Figure out ways of communicating yes and no.

Lauren remembers one especially striking moment with a client who was having a miscarriage. The client took Lauren's hand and placed it on her forehead. That moment clarified the importance of physical support during these procedures and also demonstrated how doula work creates space for clients to make these requests, verbally or nonverbally.

At Some Point, You Will Shove Your Foot in Your Mouth

And that's okay. Apologize, if necessary, which it might not be. We've found that most doulas are their own worst critics. Incorporate whatever lesson you learn into your mental filter in case the situation happens again. Forgive yourself (sooner rather than later) . . . but don't let yourself off the hook.

Your Positive Energy Matters

We all have bad days. If you're having an off day, feeling anxious or nervous about your abortion or birth shift, or feeling angry about something that happened in the clinic, it's important to bring yourself to a better emotional place *before* you see your client. Take a deep breath before you go to meet them—remember that they come first in that space. More often than not, once you are in the zone with your client, you will forget whatever was troubling you.

Part 3
Ambiguous Losses

Look Away
Mary and Sonam

Sonam points to the nail polish and looks up. She has chosen the light pink, the red, and the fuchsia.

"Those are the colors you want?" I ask.

Sonam nods yes.

I add them to our basket.

We continue along the aisles of the ninety-nine-cent store in the Bedford-Stuyvesant neighborhood of Brooklyn. "Sometimes your feet get cold during labor. Let's get some socks." We each hold up a different pair, silently searching for opinions.

This is my third afternoon with Sonam, and our communication is improving. We know how to gesture with our hands and make faces of approval or disapproval. She listens carefully to my English and sometimes responds in kind. As the hours pass, I'm becoming most familiar with Sonam's head bob from side to side. This means she isn't really sure what she wants to do, a feeling that has been growing in her alongside her unborn child.

Sonam is living down the street in a convent, a long way from her native Bhutan. She came to New York a few months earlier with her brother, mother, and father—a truck driver. Sonam is eighteen years old and eight months pregnant. I will later find out that Sonam was very much in love with the father of her child, that he left her early in the pregnancy back in Bhutan, and that this adoption is not her idea.

For now, we shop. Sonam has few belongings with her at the convent. Her room is beige, tidy, and spare, with a metal bed and a small wooden dresser. The curtains are perpetually closed, as if in a vow to let no light enter. The windows are barred as they are on every other building on this block, but here the bars seem to hold in as much as they keep out. In the resulting stillness, the convent feels unsettling in this twenty-four-hour New York City borough.

It is winter 2009. I hand a few dollars over to the cashier, and we pull our puffy coats close as we push back into the cold. The sun is shining, and Sonam and I walk arm in arm down the street, I a good foot taller. I slow my steps to match hers, glancing down with a smile. This is my first live birth as a doula, and I think I might be as expectant as Sonam. Neither of us have any idea what we are in for.

I meet with my friend Liz the following week for brunch in Greenpoint. While she tells me about her recent breakup, I pry my eyes open with caffeine, still wrecked from the previous day's stillbirth induction.

I've been living in the hospital—or so it feels—bouncing from laminaria insertions to procedures to inductions alongside Lauren. Our plan to bring on more doulas has mostly fallen short, so my weekly brunch ritual has been replaced with catching up on sleep and putting in time at my paying job at the Pro-Choice Public Education Project (PEP). I try to focus on Liz, but my cell phone sits on the table next to my coffee cup, and I check it obsessively. I'm on call for Sonam's birth, and today is zero hour.

I'm startled when it actually rings. "Hello!" It's Sonam's social worker, Ally. "Sonam's water has broken, and the ambulance is picking her up now."

"Ambulance?" I grimace at Liz. "Is she okay?"

"Yes, I think they just felt best transporting her this way." Ally sounds calm, so I try to quiet the warning bells in my head.

"Oh . . . okay. I'm heading there now—will keep in touch!" I run back to my apartment and grab my birth bag, breathless as I call Lauren. We have decided to co-doula this birth. She has attended several births before and plans to show me the ropes. We are both new to adoption and a little nervous. We've heard stories. Stories that came to us not through our years of work in the reproductive justice movement, but through the single voice of a woman I met by coincidence. One November afternoon while I was working at PEP, Marci Lieber, representing Spence-Chapin Children and Family Services—a pro-choice adoption agency committed to the rights of birth mothers—came to my office in downtown Manhattan.

In my midtwenties and smugly radical, I had never heard of Spence-Chapin, had never considered adoption much in the first place. In my abortion-centric mind at that time, adoption was what you chose if you were pro-life, and that was that. The Doula Project was still the Abortion Doula Project. While we had adapted a birthing model of care, we had yet to enter the actual birthing room.

I began to wonder how I had missed this crucial piece. Adoption accounts for less than one percent of pregnancy outcomes in the United States, a small number but one with rippling effects. As it turned out, Marci and her colleagues would become integral to bringing awareness of adoption as a broader reproductive justice issue to groups in New York and across the country. In a single conversation she gave me an education that expanded not only my own perspective but also the mission of the Doula Project.

She opened my eyes to the experience of birth mothers, particularly those on the labor and delivery floor. I learned about the time when hospital staff had created a prayer circle around the bed of a laboring mother who had "made an adoption plan" (a term preferred over the more common but categorically disempowering "gave the baby up for adoption"). I also learned about the time when a client was introduced to her baby against her wishes and about another incident where a client asked to hold her baby and was told she couldn't. I learned of mothers who were subjected to a cascade of medical interventions—Pitocin, epidural, C-section—often because they were not given the proper information on other less invasive approaches or because the staff thought they knew what was "best." Most of these stories were about the unfortunate tendencies of medical staff to do exactly the opposite of what these clients had wanted.

Still a somewhat naive and idealistic creature in the

medical community—though no stranger to stigma after years of work in abortion—I was taken aback. Surely this couldn't be the experience of all women choosing an adoption plan?

"Not all birth mothers," Marci assured me. Some have the support of family, friends, and medical professionals. It's the ones who are alone, who make their adoption and birth plans in isolation, whose entire experience of pregnancy is shrouded in secrecy and shame.

I asked Marci, "Does Spence-Chapin have doulas?" They didn't. We began to hatch a plan.

Lauren and I recognized that the clients we were serving at City Hospital didn't all fit into our original concept of "women having abortions." While they came to us through the abortion service, many didn't identify with the word. As we encountered a growing population of women experiencing miscarriages, having fetal anomalies, and opting for stillbirth inductions, our name and mission started to feel narrow and inappropriate. In a more sociopolitical sense, it felt like we were missing something key: the chance to really connect the entire spectrum of pregnancy options to each other. We could be, and should be, more open minded and all serving. Our true "mission" was to serve our clients through all their decisions from abortion to birth and everything in between.

Within a month we had partnered with Spence-Chapin and officially changed our name to the Doula Project. We would now work closely with Spence to provide educational, emotional, and physical support to their birth mothers.

Our brief run as abortion-only advocates was over. While we might have moved on and forward, our detractors would often come back to that narrow definition of who we were and what we did during that first year, ignoring the more holistic picture entirely.

When I arrive, Lauren's in the labor and delivery waiting room. "Hey!" She waves me over. "Sonam's in triage. We can meet her inside once they get a room."

The labor and delivery rooms at Bushwick Hospital are beautiful, and I feel myself relax a little. Having spent the previous day at a stillbirth induction in a particularly dated public hospital, I had expected much of the same: broken Zenith with missing remote, flickering fluorescent lights, faded gray walls, one uncomfortable chair to be shared by three people. The room we enter holds rich wooden cabinets and dressers and a rocking chair, everything accented in deep green.

Lauren and I smile at each other, feeling hopeful and energized, greeting Sonam with gentle shoulder squeezes. *This is going to be good, this is going to be better than good, it will be GREAT,* I reassure myself.

Like many mothers we would encounter at Spence-Chapin, Sonam was walking rather blindly into this experience. She had switched hospitals late in her pregnancy, after Spence helped her move out of her parents' apartment in Queens. Bushwick Hospital was the closest to her new residence. Therefore, she would go to Bushwick. Labor and delivery at Bushwick is run by a mix of obstetricians and midwives: whoever is there is who you get. During what would turn into a fifty-two-hour labor, we would see both.

Sonam's first midwife pops in the room and consults with us. "Things are looking good here! Why don't you stay out of bed, walk the hall a bit? Let's get this labor going!" She breezes out.

"Thank God they seem nice here," I whisper to Lauren. We move over to Sonam and help her out of the bed. She is stone-faced as she makes small circles around the room. I attempt to take her arm—she shakes her head, no.

As the hour passes, Sonam's OB from triage comes by to check her dilation. "Nothing so far. I would like to start her on Pitocin. I wanted to see more dilation at this point since it's been about five hours since her water broke. I'll stop back by in an hour or so."

Three physiological things need to happen for labor to begin: First, there have to be uterine contractions from the top of the uterus rather than the sides. Second, the cervix, a firm, hard muscle that feels like a tongue, needs to become soft and flat in order to dilate. And third, the baby needs to "drop," or be firmly engaged deep down in the pelvis.

Pitocin is used to create contractions and advance labor. It, like most drugs, has its uses. However, it is also used based on the assumption that birth is a linear progression of ever-greater contractions and that more contractions as fast as possible are a "good thing." The result usually is that the baby is being forced out by a drug and may become stressed by being squeezed repeatedly against an under-dilated cervix. At this moment, watching Sonam, I knew this only in theory. In retrospect, I see how it set in motion a series of near-catastrophic events.

A nurse settles Sonam into the bed, strapping her with a fetal heart monitor and a wire that offers just a few feet of pull. Sonam is literally only allowed to labor on a very tight leash. Lauren shoots me a knowing look; it's par for the course in New York City, being allowed to move only inches away from your bed in the midst of labor. Walking is a great way to relieve the discomfort of contractions and work with gravity to help the baby come down low into the pelvis, so, unfortunately, policies that prevent this can further delay and complicate labor. We ask the nurse, "Does she have to be hooked to all of this equipment so soon? She'd like to walk around a bit more." Sonam nods in agreement.

"Doctor's orders. We gotta get her induced." The nurse continues to prop and fluff pillows, barely glancing our way.

The Pitocin drip begins, and hours of slow but steady contractions follow. Day turns into night turns into day. Our time is punctuated by twelve-hour shift changes, with nurses and midwives stopping by every laboring woman's room, cheerily singing, "Good morning!" "Good evening!" like a chorus of Florence Nightingales. We find this comforting. Often the hospitals where we work are populated by jaded employees who are crushed under the weight of all of the needs of their patients in a system that is stretched too thin. They tend to skeptically regard us as novel. We hear frequently, "Doulas don't usually come here."

Lauren and I take turns massaging Sonam's legs and feet, pushing into the small of her back until our arms burn. We rock her, we dance; she meditates and takes short naps. We curl up on the cold floor with our single sheets, no pillows, stealing winks of sleep where we can. At one point Sonam offers us feedback that would become infamous during our doula careers: "You're not fanning me right."

Lauren takes on shit duty, emptying seemingly endless full yellow plastic trays into the nearby toilet as a gesture of solidarity, an olive branch, to the nurses. As Sonam's contractions become stronger, Lauren travels into the hall in search of a microwave to heat a rice pillow. She returns disheartened. It turns out the nurses aren't so pleased to have doulas on the floor after all. We have a quiet huddle.

"So what exactly happened? Are they pissed off that we're here?" I whisper, glancing over at Sonam breathing deeply with her eyes closed. I had become accustomed to our mini celebrity status in Dr. B's abortion service at City Hospital. Of course, I'd heard about the tension between doulas and nurses but had yet to experience it firsthand.

"Yes," Lauren says tearfully. "We're asking for too much." We are both exhausted. More than twenty-four hours deep, and Sonam is only a few centimeters dilated.

"I need to go cry in the bathroom." Lauren disappears to the adjoining room.

Sonam's stirring and moaning intensifies, her eyes now open and fearful. "Sonam, what is it?"

She glances at the closed door through which Lauren has departed. I reassure her, "No, everything is okay. Lauren is fine."

"I'm going to die!" Sonam cries, as Lauren comes out.

"Sonam, no, it's all right. I just got yelled at by some nurses." Lauren is red and splotchy.

"That doesn't make any sense. It's because of me," Sonam insists.

Lauren looks at me imploringly. "No, really, Sonam," I rush over to her side, "you are just fine." She stares at me hard for a moment, then closes her eyes, wincing every few seconds in pain.

"How long do you think they're gonna let her go?" I whisper over to Lauren. New York City has an infamously high C-section rate, with many hospitals reaching past 30 percent, contrasted with the World Health Organization's recommendation that only 10 to 15 percent of births should be delivered by Cesarean. Because Sonam's water broke the day before, risk of infection climbs with each hour.

Lauren puts her hand to her forehead, closing her eyes with a sigh. "I really don't know."

We go back to work as nurses stream through with bright smiles. "Epidural? Epidural?"

Epidural. Sonam gets an epidural, a needle in her spine that will, ideally, numb her from the waist down and reduce the discomfort associated with contractions. She had not intended to get one, but the pain is overwhelming and many hours of labor stretch before her. She is losing energy, both physically and emotionally. Lauren and I resist joining in this feeling; we are here to keep the bad thoughts and the loneliness at bay. But the sun-filled room we had entered the day before feels icy and hostile, and I wonder how I ever saw it any other way.

Lauren is curled up with a LUNA bar, and Sonam's epidural has taken effect. I pull the rocking chair next to Sonam and smooth her dark hair. Calmness runs through her and out into me, and I become certain that the doula-mother relationship is a symbiotic one. I wonder about Sonam's life. I have cobbled together bits of information from the social workers at Spence and from observing Sonam over the past month. Though Sonam is still a teenager, she moves with the confidence of someone much older. Her face is solemn, the rare smile always cautious. Her dark eyes appear almost black.

Her family remains a mystery to me; she has never spoken of them. Her mother is present for parts of the labor but disappears in crucial moments. Where does she go? Sonam's father knows nothing of the pregnancy, but can they really keep it a secret forever? The baby's dad is long gone, but to where and why? I will probably never know; I don't need to know much.

What I do know is that Sonam doesn't want a C-section. I know that she doesn't want to meet her baby, and that we are to make sure he is taken out of the room as quickly as possible after the birth. I know that this is her wish, and that I don't need to understand why—I can see in her eyes why. I also know that the baby is going to be called Daniel. Whose idea that is, I can't remember. I'm trying not to think too much about Daniel.

Hour forty-four, my eyes are bleary from my vigilance over the machines. *Fetal distress*, they blink. Each time the number spikes or dips, my heart goes with it. How many beats do we want? I seem to forget every few minutes. Whisperings

145

of a C-section have been floating around the last few hours. The epidural has slowed contractions; Pitocin levels have continuously increased. Everyone is worried about Daniel's heartbeat, bouncing from ninety to one hundred and sixty in a matter of seconds. Sonam continues to hum and meditate, but I can detect fear in her eyes, as if she can sense the medical staff descending.

They finally arrive and consult the monitors, the printouts, Sonam. They explain to us that they must do a C-section.

Sonam is shaking her head no: *no, she won't do the C-section.*

Her OB wearily asks what her hesitations are, pointing out that they have let her labor for many hours past their usual protocol, given her desire for vaginal birth.

Sonam continues to shake her head, eyes flashing over to Lauren and me. We move closer to the bed, attempting to provide a protective wall around her.

The OB is quick to agitate at this gesture. Her shift is ending soon, and it's up to her to make the call and get things moving into the operating room. She changes tactics, targeting Lauren and me. "Can you *please* talk to her?"

"I think there is some misunderstanding here," I begin. "Sonam is from Bhutan, and C-sections are not always safe for the mother there. Is there a way you can better explain the procedure to her, like with an interpreter?"

"Well, we can't get a Bhutanese translator this time of night." She looks at me blankly.

"There are translators available twenty-four hours a day.

There might be a delay, but you can get one." Lauren works at City Hospital and isn't buying this.

The conversation continues, the staff barely glancing at Sonam, their patient. I begin to wonder how much difference a translator will make at this point. The room has turned aggressive. The trust has been broken. Sonam begins to cry. "I understand," she tells us. There is a hush in the room as the divide deepens. It's fight night; we've already taken our corners.

"If you cannot convince her to get this C-section, then I'm going to call up hospital administration." The OB reaches for the phone.

A woman in a red suit arrives, alert and polished at 2:00 a.m., with red nails and red lipstick. She chews gum, and her smile does not reach her eyes. "I need everyone to understand that we are planning to move forward with a court-ordered C-section. This means that a judge will rule that hospital staff is allowed to perform this procedure without the mother's consent or the mother will face potential prosecution following delivery." She talks loudly but appears to be speaking to no one in particular. "This child's *life* is in danger," she finishes grandly.

We remain silent as the machines beep out Daniel's wild heartbeat. "I think you know this is best," she continues, now looking meaningfully in my direction. I realize then that they expect Lauren and me to change Sonam's mind—to make this decision for her.

Lauren and I convince the staff to find an interpreter.

The calls are made; we wait, staring at the floor, the ceiling. Finally Sonam is on the phone. There is a brief silence on the other end before the translator speaks Sonam's words: "It doesn't matter what happens to the baby because the baby is bad and doesn't have a father."

Chaos ensues. Everyone is talking at once and moving quickly, nervously around the room. A nurse that I had not noticed before says loudly in my ear: "Just because she doesn't want the baby, that doesn't mean he should die!"

I begin to feel very far away from Sonam. I float from her bedside to the farthest corner of the room, the one by the door marked EXIT. What would happen if I walked out?

"Can't you do something?" They turn to the doulas. My ignorance feels enormous. So does my guilt. What is the role of the doula when things go this horribly wrong? *I should have prepared Sonam for a C-section; I should have fought against the Pitocin, the epidural; I should have helped the doctors better understand her culture.* I think back to Marci's warnings about all the violations against birth mothers. In my arrogance, I believed I could change some of that as a first-time doula, walking as blindly into the system as my client.

"What are her options at this point?" Lauren asks.

"We do the C-section now, or she signs a refusal of care against medical advice," explains the administrator. If Sonam absolves the hospital of legal jeopardy, then what happens? The truth is that Sonam's baby could be just fine even if this went on for hours. Alternately, there is a chance that the delay would lead to some possible risk to Daniel and Sonam. The costs and benefits are not so easy to determine. We are all caught up in a vast series of decisions right now that are ostensibly about the patient's well-being, but also about legal risk. As a patient do you lose the right to your body when you enter this gray area?

The interpreter explains Sonam's options to her. Sonam looks at Lauren and me, asking not for guidance but support. We grab her hands as she speaks into the phone. "I do not want the C-section."

The OB gives a long and final sigh, defeated. "I need you to sign this form stating that you refused medical advice." Sonam puts pen to paper, and a clattering of footsteps retreat out of the room and down the hall.

Only stillness remains. Even the sounds of the monitors are in the distance, though surely Daniel's heartbeat continues to surge and drop. The violence is over.

They say that after a trauma occurs, it is best to get back into your routine as quickly as possible.

The three of us resume our day as if the past few hours had never happened. Massages and deep breaths commence. Daniel's heart rate levels out. Normalcy. There is a shift change, and a staff of fresh-faced nurses and a midwife enter the room, a warm glow ushering them through the door. "Well, everything is looking just fine here. Eight centimeters!"

Sweet sunlight creeps in, and I realize I haven't been outside in days. Lauren tells me to go get food; she has to leave for work soon. Somehow, it's Monday morning. I head toward the McDonald's across the street. The electronic menu flashes Egg McMuffins and piping hot coffee. I fall into a booth and look around, seeing students grabbing something for their walk to school and two elderly men deep in conversation while their cups steam in front of them.

Flushing Avenue is blaring and honking outside the window. *I want to go home.* Sleeplessness has never suited me well—I turn inward, become entirely selfish. What are the thoughts that run through a good doula's head, a great doula's head, in times like these? She probably thinks only of her client, not about slinking back into her own easy life, away from the noise. I fight off the overwhelming desire to stay in McDonald's and head slowly with plodding, sleepless feet toward my fears.

Back at the hospital, Lauren says her goodbyes. We have a long hug, and I don't want to let her go. It's just Sonam and me now. She is in the rocking chair where I left her, face to the window, back to me. I stoop down and entwine our hands together, her light pink fingernail polish next to my chipped black. We move back to the bed and sit in silence. I wonder if we can trust this quiet.

After a while, the midwife comes in to check Sonam's dilation. She smiles up at us. "Ladies, let's get ready—*time to push!*" We feel unprepared now that the time has arrived. Hour fifty-two. We never thought we would get to this moment. Sonam looks into my eyes, questioning: is it really happening?

I move into position, one hand in hers, another holding back her left leg. We count to ten—push!—dozens of times over. My eyes well up for what is to come, for what has already happened. As Sonam gives a final push, she pulls the sheet over her face, hands clenched tight around its corners, a pure white shield between her and her child.

The staff is in sync, with Sonam, with me. The midwife holds Daniel, cutting the cord as Sonam leans back and sobs. They rush baby Daniel out of the room. I curl myself around Sonam, holding her while tears fall. She pulls back the sheet. It is safe to look.

When I think about Sonam, I think about this old Ozzfest T-shirt I used to live in. At the last minute Ally has asked me to come up to Spence for the afternoon. Weeks have passed, the adoption has been finalized, and the adoptive parents are coming to get Daniel.

Open adoption is now the norm around the country—over half of all adoptions are fully open. This means that the birth parent has the right to keep in contact with the child, and the adoptive parent must agree to these terms. Birth parents also get to select the adoptive parent and meet them before the birth, if so desired. Photographs and letters are sent back and forth between adoptive parents and birth parents, visitations are arranged, and families are being constructed on their own terms. Sonam, however, has declined to meet Daniel's adoptive parents. The image of her lifting the white sheet to her face plays in my mind.

It starts raining as I make the long walk to First and Ninetieth from the 6 train. I knock on Ally's office door, with dripping burgundy-black hair and a giant heavy metal T-shirt. Ally doesn't seem to care; she is grateful I am here.

She rushes me to a small, overheated room. "This is Mary, Sonam's doula. She was at the birth, and she knows Daniel. She's here to help with this transition today."

"You know Sonam?" Daniel's new parents bring me into their arms, tears in their eyes. "Can you tell us about her?"

Ally offers me an encouraging look. "I'll leave you three alone for a few minutes, and then I'll bring Daniel in."

They stare at me expectantly. *What do I say? What do I say?* Sonam's birth comes rushing back to me . . . the burning in my muscles, the woman in the red suit, Sonam's big, watery eyes. It hits me: I don't know where she is now. Is she back with her family, her father never the wiser, her mother quietly frantic? What are Sonam's memories of the birth? Is she at work, out in the world, sitting alone in her apartment? How many times a day does she think of Daniel?

I refocus—I am overwhelmed by the hope in their eyes, their frozen smiles, as if I am the only window they have into this woman who has given them their most precious gift. I might be. "It's wonderful to meet you," I take a deep breath. I tell them the good parts—about her quiet strength during long contractions, about us rocking back and forth in each other's arms, and holding hands in the sun-filled streets of Bed-Stuy. I don't mention the hospital staff, our fear about Daniel's health, or the confusion and anger in Sonam's face. I'm not sure why. Maybe I don't want to ruin the moment. Maybe I don't want it to be part of their story, of Daniel's story. Maybe I am protecting Sonam.

The meeting is over, and I step outside, stunned. I'm learning that this is what it is to be a doula: to be allowed into someone's life at its most crucial point, to understand that it's a moment in time. Then, you are left with only the memory, and you have to figure out where to put it.

Back up Ninetieth Street, I don't bother with an umbrella. I think the rain might save me. Tears mix with raindrops as I blink up at the sky. One day Daniel will ask about his birth mom. His parents will tell him that she is a brave and beautiful woman. They know this because a frizzy-haired girl in a giant Ozzfest T-shirt told them one stormy afternoon.

Open and Closed
Lauren, Mary, and Kiya

It's a hot, sticky day in 2009 just as spring is turning to summer. We ditch work early and make our way uptown, exhausted as usual. Our recent catapult into full-spectrum doula work has us running. In addition to providing abortion care, we now attend births too. Today, we are headed to the Spence-Chapin offices to meet our newest birth client, Kiya.

Six months after the Doula Project's maiden volunteer training, we continue to be the organization's only two birth doulas, with four other volunteers now assisting in the abortion clinic. When birth clients are referred, we use a co-doula system, a practice that ensures that our clients have support from both of us throughout their labor and delivery. Because our birth clients are often alone during their pregnancies and deliveries, we have found that they prefer the extra person in the room. Therefore, we make it our business for both of us to be there.

We co-doula for our clients but for ourselves as well: we

are there to support one another, too. We have found that because we are working with clients whose experiences often go unconsidered in traditional doula trainings—those having stillbirth inductions or creating adoption plans—we run the risk of feeling isolated if we work alone. It's not so much that "no one can understand what we are doing," it's more that we are unsure of how to process it all—the experience itself and where we "belong" in someone else's story. We still don't know how being doulas, especially full-spectrum doulas, is going to shape us. We just know that we need to have another person in the room who sees "it," whether it's the threat of a court-ordered C-section, a client who screams inconsolably for six hours straight during her stillbirth, or the moment when the deceased baby is delivered and it feels like there is only a sucking vacuum of silence. We don't know who to talk to or how to talk about it, so we talk to each other, often over spanakopita and french fries in the requisite Greek diners within the New York City public hospital system.

Kiya is one in a string of clients this spring who has come to us with an adoption plan. Her social worker has filled us in on the bits of her life we need to know in order to fulfill our role. Kiya is living at Inwood House, a group home for pregnant and parenting teenagers who are in the foster care system. Independent, determined, and a little stubborn, Kiya often has to fend for herself. Though her family is large, she doesn't have anyone to depend on. Her mother passed away when she was younger, her father is not especially involved in her life, and she is only tangentially in touch with her siblings. She is a good student, plays the saxophone in the school band, and works a salaried job for the New York Census Bureau doing payroll. Kiya has many friends but maintains a safe distance from most people. She needs to ensure her privacy, especially now that she is pregnant.

Today, and in the weeks that follow, Kiya shares her story with us.

She became pregnant just as she was entering her senior year, filling out college applications and making plans for a new life away from New York. She wanted to become either an astronomer or a lawyer, maybe both. At first the thought that she could be pregnant was so foreign to her that she didn't even consider it. She used protection every time she had sex. And anyway, she was anemic, so missing a period or two wasn't abnormal. A baby was unfathomable for her and what she wanted for her future. Never mind the fact that the would-be father dropped off the face of the earth as soon as she told him she was pregnant. What was she supposed to do?

She made an appointment to have an abortion at a clinic that offered both family planning services and prenatal care. She approached this abortion as one might approach a surprise bungee jumping trip—with great apprehension. She didn't *want* an abortion. She didn't *want* to be there, young and pregnant and vulnerable. She felt guilty and frustrated with herself, with her boyfriend-turned-sperm-donor, with the fact that she was living proof that condoms aren't 100 percent effective. She sat in the crowded waiting room, resigning herself to her decision. *It's necessary*, she thought.

When she was finally summoned back to the exam room, she realized that the clinic had made a mistake—she had been scheduled for a prenatal care appointment instead of a consultation for an abortion. In busy clinics serving multiple patient needs, this mistake is not uncommon, if also unfortunate. When Kiya tells this story now, people often openly speculate that she was bullied into having the baby by a clinic with an antiabortion agenda, although she feels that it was indeed an error in appointment.

She was ready to correct the clinic, but then . . . she didn't. At the time she couldn't explain it, but she sat through the entire prenatal care appointment. She didn't say anything when she was scheduled for the next one either. She found that she just kept going until she realized that she didn't want an abortion after all.

Now Kiya speaks more plainly about what compelled her to go to all of those prenatal care appointments: "Guilt," she says. "Today I don't have that kind of guilt, I would [have an abortion if I needed to]. But being so young I had that guilt."

Okay, so she knew that, regardless of the reasons, she wasn't going to have an abortion. But now what? Her family wasn't very supportive—"they still aren't very supportive"—and she had no idea where to start. She knew she didn't want to give up her career goals, and she wasn't sure she was ready to parent. She began to tepidly consider an adoption plan.

Less than one percent of pregnancies result in adoption, and much of the conversation around adoption has been appropriated by antiabortion activists. This all works together to create a perfect storm of inaccessibility and confusion so that when people consider making adoption plans, finding clear answers can feel impossible. Kiya quickly learned that it's not easy to uncover resources that are centered on the needs of birth parents. She didn't have many places to turn, so she went to her high school guidance counselor. He perked up when he heard her adoption plans; he had friends in Florida who were looking to adopt a baby.

When Kiya spoke to this couple, she was immediately disconcerted. They told her up front that they had lawyers on their side. They were requesting a "closed adoption," which meant that Kiya, as the birth parent, would relinquish all of her rights to communicate with her child and that any records with information about her would be sealed as far as the baby was concerned. She would never be able to see the child, and she would never receive pictures or updates. He wouldn't know anything about her and would never be able to find her, even if he wanted to. In fact, the couple said that they planned to keep the adoption a secret from the child. He would never even know that he was adopted. That's why, in part, they were trying to make sure that they would adopt a baby that was African American like them.

Kiya was unnerved by this and took some time to think about it. She wanted an open adoption in which both parties could negotiate the boundaries of her relationship with the child. Adoption is extremely complex and criminally simplified in popular and political culture. Studies show that everyone tends to fare better in open adoptions: birth parents, adoptive parents, and, most of all, the children who are adopted. Open communication reduces the stigma around adoption for everyone—it's not perfect, but it's much healthier than hiding an adoption. But that wasn't what this couple wanted, and Kiya felt like she didn't have many other options.

Two weeks passed, and Kiya decided that she would do it. She felt relieved, excited even, to have the "Yes I will" conversation with them. This was going to be the answer to all of the grief of this pregnancy. They would get the baby they wanted, the baby would get loving parents, and Kiya could continue down the path she was on. She knew it would be hard, but this seemed like the best option.

She called the couple on the subway ride home from school.

"Oh, we already have another baby lined up," they told her. "Sorry."

It was as if all the air left her lungs. She felt wooden as the conversation went on and, surprisingly, jealous.

They offered to adopt Kiya's baby, too. "Like twins," they said.

Kiya then realized, "They just wanted a baby. I don't think they cared by whom. They wanted a baby that could pass for theirs."

She was irrelevant to them. What she wanted had never mattered, so much so that they were able to make a decision without any regard for her, her pregnancy, or the sheer impact they would have on her life. The only thing that mattered to them was that they wanted the baby she was carrying—so long as it would be convenient for them.

At this point she was very far along, about seven months. Now she couldn't have an abortion even if she wanted to. The fact that Kiya was trying to do things independently made her all the more defenseless. She had absolutely no one to protect her and no idea who to ask for help. Without a knowledgeable institution on her side, like her school, a lawyer, or an adoption agency, she became very vulnerable, very quickly.

She moved into a dark place inside, going through the motions of her life while feeling heavy and lost, dragging herself to school every morning, spacing out in class, wandering around alone each night. Eventually she was invited to live at Inwood House, where she would at least have a safe place to land for a while. There she was put in touch with Spence-Chapin, the organization that would ultimately guide Kiya toward making a decision that she could be comfortable with. At Spence-Chapin, the ball would be in her court. She would choose the adoptive family, and she would choose the terms of the adoption: Open or closed? And if open, would that mean pictures and emails sometimes or would it mean visits? Kiya would even have a "grace period" of thirty days after the baby was born to reconsider becoming a parent.

Kiya would see her social worker, Joann, once every week or two until all aspects of the adoption plan were settled. She remembers now:

I loved Spence, I loved Joann, she was wonderful and patient. [It was] a very good experience. She didn't put pressure on me either way. If I wanted to go through with [the adoption plan] she supported me, and if I didn't, she supported me as well. She gave me resources. I remember talking to her every week. She was kind of like a counselor to me. We talked about the process, what the severance of rights looks like, the different types of adoption that happen.

After a few meetings, Joann contacted Mary and Lauren. She thought Kiya was the perfect candidate for a doula.

Initially Kiya is skeptical of the idea of a doula. "I didn't understand what birth was like at all," she says now. "I thought it was like TV, like you go in with an overwhelming amount of pain, and you're screaming, and you have to get an epidural because [the] pain is inhumanly unendurable. So I thought I would have to get an epidural and just lay there, and then the doctor [would do] something special, and the baby [would be] born, and what I had to do was minimal. Or I would have to have a C-section. I thought that was normal."

One day, Kiya sees one of the other residents at Inwood House go into labor in the middle of the night. It's the first time Kiya has seen anyone in labor, and the mother-to-be is having a rough time. She also has a doula.

Less impressed with the doula than the amount of discomfort her housemate is in, Kiya realizes that having extra support is probably a good idea. She recalls, "I didn't really understand what you could do that would make a difference. What would the doula do? You were telling me, but I was like, 'Eh, we'll see.'"

Though not completely convinced of the magic of doulas, Kiya wants to be prepared. Beyond seeing the potential need for doula support, Kiya also begins to take an interest in natural birth. Between watching a beautiful birthing video at Inwood House—a woman in an adobe home, squatting in her garden, surrounded by family, calm—and having the trademark Lauren-and-Mary unsentimental childbirth education during a prenatal visit, she is inspired to do research on natural birth. "I was like, 'Whoa is that what that's like? It can be that way?'" She remembers, "I decided I didn't want a passive role in giving birth, especially if I was going to consider adoption."

We begin to see Kiya regularly to talk about birth, the adoption, and her life. A lot of our meetings happen over pizza, in public spaces, where people move away from us the second the phrase "mucous plug" comes up in conversation. "You'll know your mucous plug is gone because it will look like your vagina sneezed!" (Thank you Antoinette Leonard Jean-Charles for that useful description, which has been passed on to countless clients and doulas.)

She tells us that she has chosen a name for the baby. "Vladimir," she says proudly.

A name with a lot of character: a big statement. It's something she feels strongly about. She is sure that Vladimir will be her baby's name.

We talk about school, where she is living, her favorite foods.

"I really miss sushi," she confides. "I'm a pescatarian." Now she has a newfound appreciation for burgers and fries.

"How long have you both been doulas?" she wants to know.

"Lauren's been an active doula for several years, but I'm mostly just starting out. I've been to a few births with Lauren," Mary says.

Kiya nods thoughtfully. "Well, it's my first time giving birth. It will be special for both of us."

She is curious about us. She asks us questions, softly inquisitive about who we are and why we decided to become doulas. We talk shop a lot—"this is birth, this is how we can help"—but being invited to attend someone's birth is an intimate honor, so we all take the time to get to know one another. We don't want to create hierarchies when we don't have to.

Through the chaos of this makeshift childbirth education, Kiya is wrapping up high school and going to Spence-Chapin regularly to plan for what will happen after the birth. It's time to choose a family to adopt, or potentially adopt, her baby.

First Kiya looks through a huge binder filled with adoptive parents with basic descriptions: a happy picture, an overview of who they are, what they do, why they want to adopt a child. From there, Kiya narrows down her options and looks at the "parent books," which prospective adoptive parents create to show birth parents who they are in greater detail. Some of the books are ornate with intricate binding, lavish paper, and glossy images. People include pictures of themselves at their happiest, of their families and other children, if they have them. It is an opportunity for them to show their best selves to the birth parents. Doulas and social workers occasionally joke that *we* would like to be adopted by these families.

Kiya chooses a single gay man named George as the adoptive parent for her baby. He is an artist, appears responsible, and lives comfortably. Kiya admires the life he lives and thinks, *I would want him to adopt me too.*

They meet in the Spence office. George brings a small puppet for the baby with him, for when he is born. Kiya is transparent about where she is at—that she is probably going to go through with the adoption, but there is definitely a possibility that she will want to parent. She also tells him that she plans to breast-feed, at least for a little while.

He is very understanding. Kiya wonders whether another birth mother will choose him if she doesn't go through with the adoption plan.

She tells George that she intends to name the baby Vladimir.

"*Vladimir?*" he says with surprise.

Kiya nods proudly.

"What about something softer, like Niall?" George suggests.

Nope. That's not what she wants. They agree to keep talking about it and part ways. *His name is Vladimir,* she thinks.

Kiya tells us this story during one of our requisite pizza dates. At this point she is hugely pregnant but still traveling all over the city to doctors' appointments, school, and Medicaid offices. To add insult to injury, she has to switch doctors late in the pregnancy, ostensibly for insurance reasons. She remembers now, "When I told [the doctor] it was an insurance problem, he told me, 'You're gonna have residents who don't know what they are doing' and he told me I should pay him in cash."

164

Horrified and unable to even consider paying her doctor cash to manage her birth, she switches to a group of family practice providers. That's when she makes a nauseating discovery about her first doctor: "[He] was going on vacation when Vlad was supposed to be born," she says now, "and I remember he put in his notes that I had a really low-lying placenta that was covering the birth canal. When I finally changed doctors, they did an emergency sonogram . . . and the placenta was nowhere in the way. So I thought about why he said that . . . maybe it was so he could do the C-section, go on his vacation, and get paid."

Kiya has likely dodged a bullet by having to switch doctors. We take the hospital tour with her. She likes the residents at the new practice. They are young, patient, and exuberant about their work. We walk (waddle) through the halls with a group of other very pregnant people, all joking that it is like being on the set of *March of the Penguins*. At this point, Kiya is extremely close to her due date. She wins the prize for "Most Pregnant Mom" on the tour. We even mention playfully that she could go into labor during the tour, if she wants to.

Kiya has become committed to having an unmedicated, vaginal delivery, but we can't help but worry whether a hospital birth is conducive to that. She tells her doctors about her desires for a natural labor. They are supportively blasé about it. "Okay, great, whatever," they say.

At this point there isn't much to do except help Kiya plan to labor at home for as long as possible—this is the key to reducing the risk of extra medical interventions, as many doulas can attest. We would learn through experience that by the time we saw many of our clients, their birth plans were often pretty settled and often very limited. We aren't going to stress Kiya out by making her review her options for other doctors. But we do keep an eye out for red flags. Call it "doula skepticism."

Kiya's due date comes and goes. We try to keep her calm. Lauren and Kiya speak daily. "Hey, how are you? Still pregnant?"

Kiya's doctors get anxious and start using the *i* word: *induction*. With several unfortunate induction-related birth experiences—like Sonam's—under our belts, we are hoping that Kiya might be able to avoid the same fate. We share tips and tricks to induce labor at home: "Here's a recipe from a restaurant in North Carolina that claims its eggplant parmesan is foolproof for starting labor," and "If you can't do acupuncture, massage the tender spot that's four finger-breadths above your inner ankle."

None of it works. Kiya finally has a conversation with her doctors. "If you don't give birth by the end of this week, we are going to induce," they tell her.

She calls Lauren in a panic. Lauren is at a Starbucks, interviewing people who would become part of the 2009 cohort of Doula Project volunteers and would eventually join our leadership circle and make the organization what it is today. Mary is doing the same in Brooklyn.

"What am I supposed to do now?" Kiya says, exasperated.

Lauren tells her about castor oil, a powerful bowel irri-

166

tant that is often a potent way to start labor. "It's messy but effective."

"What does that mean?"

"Diarrhea, mostly. Sometimes vomiting. And sometimes both at once." Pause. "You sure you don't want to give it a couple more days to see if labor doesn't start on its own?"

Kiya sighs. She isn't sure. She needs to think about it.

A few hours later she finds herself mixing six ounces of castor oil—double the usual dose—with apple juice. She calls Lauren at 5:00 a.m. (what we have found is the "witching hour" for people to go into labor) to announce that this is it: she's going to have the baby today.

"*Six ounces?* Oh, God. Are you okay?"

She's okay enough, except that her contractions are happening in a bum-rush, one right after the other. She manages her labor by pacing around her house for a solid four hours. Finally, we make plans to meet at the hospital. Lauren's mind flashes to her overscheduled day; it's the one day during Kiya's on-call period that she won't be able to attend the birth. Lauren calls Mary to coordinate passing off the birth bag filled with massage oil, sippy straws, tennis balls, and all of the rest of the doula accoutrements.

We meet in the hospital lobby, drink coffee, and set up a game plan. Mary refills the birth bag with Vitamin Water and LUNA bars, the official meal of on-call doulas and their clients. She also throws in some celebrity dish magazines for good measure. Lauren laments the timing of it all. It's the heartache of doula work, especially when you're trying to balance it with a new job or freelance commitments, to spend so much time with a client only to miss the crucial moment of the labor and birth. But given the track record we've had at previous births, we know it is just as likely that the labor will still be happening once Lauren is off work. Work is at City Hospital about ten blocks away, and she makes plans to take a very extended lunch break.

This is the first labor that Mary will attend that she is actually looking forward to, after two stillbirth inductions and Sonam's disastrous threatened-court-order C-section. She is nervous but excited. Everything is happening quickly, but given her previous birth experiences she is anticipating a long day and night.

Kiya arrives at the hospital with her friend, Monica, just as Lauren is leaving. She is draped in a long white dress covered in blue and green flowers and wears a scarf around her head. Composed as ever, she announces that her water broke in the cab on the way downtown—a classic New York story that gets chuckles out of all the nurses and doctors.

Mary immediately goes into doula mode. Kiya is in active labor and experiencing intense pain, mostly located in her back. While they wait to be admitted to triage—step one of the admissions process—Kiya walks up and down the hall with Mary in tow. Mary hands her water to drink between contractions. Her contractions are about a minute and a half apart and thirty seconds long—she is getting close to the end.

There is no room available for Kiya, so in the middle of the waiting area, Mary administers a pain-relief technique she learned in birth doula training. She has Kiya lean against a chair while she gets onto her hands and knees and pushes her palms into Kiya's lower back. After thirty minutes of this they move to triage. Contractions continue to come hard and fast, and Mary and Kiya take their stances.

Mary remembers moments from her lackluster birth doula training, where she was made to feel inadequate by a dour and possibly antiabortion trainer. Now, she realizes, she knows what she is doing . . . partially because Kiya is so supportive of *her* as a doula, grateful for the pressure on her lower back and all of the kindness that goes along with Mary's care. Kiya now describes a lot of what Mary did during her birth as an act of translation:

> She knew exactly what I needed. She knew when I needed water, she knew when I needed a snack. She would advocate for me. I was so glad I had her there. I didn't have a support system, I didn't have a bunch of people meeting me at the hospital. Even to this day when I have back pain I think, "I wish I had Mary here for one of her massages, I'm gonna go back for her massage."

A nurse comes in and out, attempting to hook Kiya up to fetal heart and contraction monitors. She asks Kiya to lie on her side to better monitor the baby's heart, making it hard for Mary to give her back the amount of pressure she needs. Luckily, lying on her side aids in rotating the baby and the back pain slowly fades.

Finally, the resident doctor consults the data from Kiya's monitors and checks her dilation: in a blur of less than an hour, she has gone from four centimeters to nine centimeters. They rush to find a space for Kiya to deliver the baby. Kiya expresses the urgency of getting a room by vomiting the burger and fries from the night before all over triage. They are quickly transferred.

This is the first time that Mary will attend a birth that isn't medicalized; it's the natural labor that Kiya wanted. The doctors prepare the bed for Kiya to begin pushing. She takes control immediately, asking the doctors why she has to lie down to give birth. They respond by bringing in a squat bar for her to hold on to while she pushes. She is attuned to her body, pushing during strong contractions.

Lauren walks in at this moment, holding flowers, expecting to hang out for a couple of hours on her lunch break. Instead she joins in on the chanting. "Push! Push!"

Thirty minutes later he is here: Vladimir.

Kiya lies there exhausted and happy.

Lauren comments, "Best lunch break ever."

We look over at Kiya and at each other, relieved, the shadows of our last few births fading a little to the background. We both needed this happy moment too.

Vladimir is in his newborn bed getting warmed up. Her friend Monica cuts the umbilical cord with the nurse, and Mary goes with Vladimir to be weighed. Like many first-time mothers, Kiya has to be stitched, a small disadvantage of having a fast labor and a baby with a perfectly round head. When Vladimir returns to the room, the nurse swaddles him in soft blankets and hands him to Kiya. She puts him to her breast, holding his tiny head up. His mouth opens and closes, trying to latch. Kiya looks into his eyes: he is her beautiful baby.

We are in the full heat of summer: training new doulas, rushing in and out of the clinic on a daily basis, checking in with former clients. We keep in constant touch with Kiya.

After her delivery, Kiya first considers working with Spence-Chapin's interim care program, where babies can be placed for up to thirty days to give birth mothers time to make preparations. Then, she decides she will bring Vladimir home with her to see if she can handle parenting. She takes to breast-feeding, lovingly changes diapers, learns to nap when he naps, watches with pride as friends and housemates fuss over him. Surrounded by the group of new young mothers at Inwood House, she becomes inspired. Her confidence in herself grows. More than anything, she knows she can't be without Vladimir. She asks Joann to inform George that she will not be choosing adoption for her son after all.

We travel to Inwood House to visit Kiya. We wander through the Bronx in a rainstorm, completely lost, calling Kiya who laughs and helpfully gives us directions. When we arrive, Lauren gives Vladimir a diaper change while Mary and Kiya dive into conversation and a huge bucket of Doritos.

"I'm working on your birth story now," Mary says, mouth full of the bright-orange chips. "It's the first one I've written." Often, part of the doula service is writing a birth story for the client so they can have a documented memory of their experience.

"I can't wait to read it," Kiya says, reaching for Vladimir as Lauren joins them on the couch.

Kiya thinks back to her early days with Vladimir now. "When you give birth, you have this overwhelming sense of love. So I had this overwhelming emotion toward this kid, and I was scared to not know what his future would be." She stays in New York City for another year after Vladimir's birth; she savors that time. Eventually she moves across the country to start school at the University of Arizona.

Vladimir turned six at the end of June. The decision Kiya made to parent him has not been without struggle: school, work, single motherhood, no familial safety net, and very little money. "What no one tells you," she says, "is that having a newborn is easy, really easy. It's not until they're older that it gets difficult. When they're about two. For me that was hard. Finding childcare . . . day-to-day life was difficult."

She puts one foot in front of the other and hopes for the best. There was a long time, until Vladimir was three or four, when she regretted not going through with the adoption—mostly because she has been alone. "The most difficult thing wasn't Vlady himself," she says, "it wasn't taking care of him. It was not having a support system. Because it was just me."

She remains passionate about natural birth, seeing her own as one of the most important moments of her life, not only because of her son but because she saw a profound, unmatchable power in herself. It was a significant turning point. "If I have one good memory, it would have to be Vladimir's birth," she says. "But it wouldn't have been as good without a doula. It wouldn't have been the experience I wanted it to be."

We would continue to doula for young mothers, supporting them through adoption plans or plans to parent. We still look to Kiya and her story as a guiding light, a symbol of the truly symbiotic nature of our work, the graceful exchange at its best. As Mary told Lauren on that day more than six years ago, "Kiya's birth has made me addicted—I am so excited to be a doula."

We cherish these moments; sometimes we don't realize how important it is to be boundlessly joyful.

How to Talk to the Press

A mini chapter—featuring other doula organizations from around the country—on lessons we have learned (mostly the hard way) about working with the press. This chapter is geared toward people hoping to start their own full-spectrum doula groups.

Anticipate the Questions

To put it quite simply, this work is not easy to talk about. Even with the most thoughtful, well-intentioned journalists, the final write-up often resembles something like sensationalism. Especially in the beginning, when the abortion doula was such a new concept, the nuances were difficult for reporters to grasp.

We recommend preparing in advance when speaking to the press. Develop a mock interview and run through a "rehearsal." Put together a handful of stories that you would be comfortable sharing and that aren't exploitative to your clinic or client. Research how other organizations that you respect have talked about this issue.

"Anticipate the inevitable questions—such as the classic 'How can you support *birth* and *abortion*?'—and know your reproductive justice stats," suggests full-spectrum doula Janna Blair Slack in Lane County, Oregon, founder of the LA Doula Project.

"Be honest, be emotional, and humanize the work we do," suggests Nafeesa Dawoodbhoy of the SPIRAL Collective in Minneapolis, Minnesota. "Abortion encompasses the human experience like no other. It is an intersection of autonomy, loss, and pain in a highly contentious political battleground."

Develop a Media Policy with Talking Points

It is important for your organization to develop a media policy that outlines effective talking points as well as messages to avoid. Isolate points that pay particular attention to the weightier, more difficult questions such as those about second trimester abortion. When in doubt, try to answer every question with your prepared talking points.

Train all media representatives in your organization and have a designated media coordinator to help guide doulas through potential interviews and tough questions. Talk to other full-spectrum doula organizations to see what kind of policies they have in place.

Be Aware of Your Own Interviewing Anxieties

If you are new to speaking publicly about full-spectrum doulas, your nerves may be on edge. Anxiety can make you more likely to stray from your core message or leave out crucial content that should have been included. Being aware of your own anxiety can help you come up with strategies for calming yourself and giving the best interview you can.

Be Proactive

Seek out news publications instead of having them seek you out. Pitch your own stories and even your own writing. You know the work best and can exercise better control over the content this way. But remember, even if you are writing the piece, the editor still has final say on the content—and the title!

Research How the Publication Represents Other Difficult Issues

Before agreeing to an interview with a publication, we recommend you research other articles they have published that cover similar issues. This is a great way to look into the political leanings of the publication and determine if you will be comfortable with them writing about your work.

Interview the Journalist

You have the right to ask journalists about their backgrounds—both about their writing on reproductive justice and their personal feelings on the issue at hand. You can also ask what angle they plan to take and which people and organizations they plan to interview. Remember, though, journalists are often at the mercy of their editor or publication and don't always have a say over the final printed product. Still, you can ask that they confirm any quotes or attributed paraphrases with you.

Always Protect Your Work and Clients First

The press often asks us for access to our clinics and clients. We have been generous in the past, and it has not always been to our benefit.

Remember: You Don't Have to Answer Every Question

While it might not always seem like it, interviews are on your terms, and you don't have to answer questions you aren't comfortable with. We often use phrases like: "That's confidential information" or "Can I get back to you about that? I need to consult with my team."

"The advice I would give is to be honest and keep the details of people's lives confidential," says Poonam Dreyfus-Pai. "[The] media loves to make stories feel more fantastical or dramatic than they might actually be, but these are people's actual lives. They're not just stories for people to consume."

Remember: You Don't Have to Talk about
Second Trimester Abortion

Make it clear to the interviewer that you work across the spectrum of pregnancy options and want to talk about all the work you engage in. We've started doing this, and journalists are usually quite compliant. They don't want to make enemies; they just want a good story. So give a good story on your own terms.

Of course, sometimes journalists will contact you to talk about a specific aspect of your work based on the angle of the article they are writing. As always, it is up to you what message you want to share with them.

Make Sure the Conversation Is Recorded

Ask the journalist to tape the interview. It's important to be quoted accurately. The way we discuss this work is nuanced and not easily accessible, even to seasoned journalists with good intentions. A tape recorder—or the Voice Memos app on your phone—can help ensure that your words are not misinterpreted or paraphrased in a way that does not represent the work as you planned.

Know When and Where to Speak to the Press . . . and When and Where Not To

Be wary of inviting press into your homes and training sites or anywhere you might be inclined to let your guard down and discuss your work in a less professional or prepared manner. Since many doula groups don't have offices, we have found it's most neutral to meet journalists in spaces like coffee shops, restaurants, or parks.

We once made the mistake of inviting a young journalist writing for a major publication to a training session. As this was training for medical students on the doula model of care, we were free to be more explicit than usual. The students were already knowledgeable, and we cut to the chase more quickly when it came to discussing procedures, particularly second trimester abortions.

Unfortunately, this turned out to be a mistake and was a huge lesson learned for us. The journalist published a story that discussed the intimate details of second trimester abortion without context. Soon the antichoice movement was publishing articles such as: "Abortion Doula Founder

Admits Those Pictures Pro-Life Activists Flash Are Real!" "Abortion Doulas Comfort Frightened Women as They Kill Their Babies," and "I Always Knew There was Something Terribly Wrong with the Doula Project."

Be Willing to Give Up Opportunities

You don't have to accept every press request that comes your way. If you feel that the conversation is going in a negative direction or that you have to compromise your work, you can always decline.

We began an interview process with a major Canadian radio station and then we chose to cancel for several reasons. First, they asked us three different times in the pre-interview if we had had abortions. Next, they rescheduled our interview at the last minute (not a deal breaker; this is common with "human-interest stories"). Finally, they formatted our segment in a way that would pit us against another feminist who had just released a book about abortion as a social good, casting us as an organization with the stance that abortion is always a tragedy. We ultimately decided that, while we would miss out on major exposure, we weren't comfortable with the approach they were taking to our work.

Know the Article May Be Written without Your Input

Often journalists will ask someone else to talk about the work if you refuse; they have a story they want to write and will likely make it happen. If you know there is going to be an article about full-spectrum doulas, it can benefit you to engage with the press. Have a voice. Get out in front of the story.

Be Prepared to Be Misquoted

You will likely be misquoted at some point, particularly if you are working with less experienced journalists. Misquotes are an inevitability if you do enough interviews. If you are misquoted and it's egregious, request that an editor's correction be posted. Otherwise, try to brush it off—you may be the only one who noticed it.

Once when we were featured in an article in the *New York Observer*, several quotes were misattributed, taken grossly out of context, and paraphrased without consideration for the delicacy of the subject. We called the editor and requested certain quotes be changed as we felt they were dangerous to our work. While we did not get all the quotes removed, they did concede a few of our points.

It's Inevitable . . . the Antichoice Movement Is Coming

If you work in abortion care, and especially if you speak publicly about that work, it is likely that you're going to receive attention from antichoice activists. In fact, as we go to print, clinics around the country are under attack. If someone from the antichoice movement targets you, make sure you keep your doulas and clinics safe. We recommend that you do not publish contact information that would identify your doulas or publicly list your clinic sites unless you clear it with them beforehand.

Don't engage with the antichoicers online. They will write inflammatory or inaccurate statements about your work and about you. And some love to make it personal.

One of our first interviews with the *Brooklyn Ink* led us straight into the open arms of the antichoice movement. At the time, the Doula Project address was Mary's home address and had been published on our website for donation purposes. It was quickly deleted. For good measure, the journalist had also included a physical description of Lauren (which was luckily inaccurate). Suddenly, we were popping up on dozens of antichoice blogs and newsletters. Some notable headlines included, "Abortion Doulas Are Wolves in Sheeps' Clothing" and "Dr. Frankenstein's Medicine Show."

Have a Sense of Humor and a Friend to Laugh With

No matter how great or thoughtful an article is, you may have at least one mortifying quote. Remember that you are likely the only person who will notice it. The day the story comes out, if it's with a major news source or if you are really stressing, get together with a friend or doula colleague so you can cringe or laugh together. It's how we've made it through some humiliating times.

Remember: The Press Can Be a Wonderful Tool for Promoting Your Work

In order to reach new audiences and gain widespread momentum for your work, cultivating relationships with different news outlets and reporters is key. Being open and accessible while sticking to organizational boundaries and talking points is a skill that will ultimately benefit your organization.

Part 4

A Crisis of Self-Care

Too Much to Give
Symone and Carol

There is no easy way to escape the March blues in New York City. The sky is forever hazy over dirty, cracked snow. Eyes behind dark glasses search for a sun that never fully shows itself. Hands like icicles still reach in pockets for frayed gloves bought six months ago. Bodies move rigidly, corpselike in tightly drawn coats. They say spring is coming, but maybe it really isn't this time. March keeps going, making a month feel like a year.

Symone sits in a waiting room at West Side Hospital, clutching a Women, Infants, and Children (WIC) pamphlet. It's been in her hand for a while now, wedded to her thin fingers, and she's read its contents several times over. The folded paper provides her with nourishment, and she clings to it. She doesn't put it down because she doesn't want to look up. If she looks up, she knows what she will see: a room full of people who, just like her, don't want to be here.

Her heart clenches at her own thought: *How could I not want to be here?*

She shifts restlessly in her chair, the itch of agitation crawling through her. She finally glances sideways at the older woman and young boy next to her. They've been here as long as Symone. The woman's lined and tired face makes it difficult to determine whether she is mother or grandmother to the boy, who obediently stares at the wall where a television should be. As Symone takes a closer look, the woman gracelessly pushes her forefinger into her nostril and digs around.

Holding back a groan, Symone jumps from her seat. She pulls out her phone and flips through its screens, pacing, looking for any distraction. A few months ago, she would have called her partner, leaving the WIC pamphlet still tucked into its plastic holder. But they broke up, a loss that punctuates Symone's recent hollowness.

She hovers near the waiting room entrance, tugging on the sleeves of her three-quarter-length cardigan. It's 3:00 p.m., and she doesn't know where to go. She doesn't want to be here, but she also doesn't want to be upstairs. Upstairs is labor and delivery, where Carol, her client, currently breathes and moans toward the birth of her child. The small room is already filled to capacity with Symone's co-doula, Erica, and her client's partner, Jason. An intimate circle. Symone was up there in the early afternoon, cycling in and out with Erica due to the hospital's two-person-maximum policy, a common feature of New York City birthing life.

While the delivery room itself is poorly designed—awkwardly crammed with metal furniture, humming machines, and lights that are better left off, she has always found peace in the view through the picture window. It reveals expansive co-op buildings, the mushroom-colored brick of the city college, bright yellow cabs rushing through the streets below. Though a few avenues away from the water, Symone could close her eyes and feel its cool, cleansing quality floating toward her on the breeze. "One day we might be able to afford this view," she joked with Carol during early labor, as they imagined the lives of the residents of the Upper West Side. They projected lives of privilege and elegance. Lives in which they didn't have to engage in the hopelessness that takes over at the end of winter.

The inside of the hospital room tells a story of a different kind of life. It's a story that has consumed Symone for the better part of four months, since she started working with Carol during her second trimester. It's a story that has merged with the dozens of other stories that Symone has taken in over the past few years—yet it stands distinct in its immediacy. It's the story of a pregnant mom of four who has recently returned to an abusive partner, the father of her baby.

Symone and Erica first met Carol just before the holidays in December 2012. The three women sat sunken into red vinyl booths at a diner on Ninety-Sixth and Broadway. It was 7:00 p.m. and pitch black outside—a stark contrast to the bright lights reflecting off the plastic menus, causing them to squint. Symone ordered her usual hot tea, abiding by her own rule to never get food in case her clients could not afford it. She pulled out her notebook and the standard Doula Project birth contract, pen poised. She was excruciatingly detailed in her note-taking. The initial prenatal meetings tended to lay out the intricacies of the birth plan and any provider concerns. These meetings were mostly straightforward in their content to a relatively seasoned doula like Symone.

The diner was packed, and they were in the center of the madness. Customers squeezed by to get to the bathrooms and crowded into the booths surrounding them. But in spite of how public the space was, Carol boomed out the intimacies of her life, going back twenty years in time. As she listened, Symone drew closer, her adopted doula stance taking shape. She pushed her dark-framed glasses up—an almost neurotic motion she has established to combat her tiny nose. She stretched her swanlike neck earnestly toward Carol as if she were leaning into her, trying to understand her. She felt somewhat dazzled by Carol who stood five foot nine and broad, with a stunning face and regal carriage. Her elegance was powerful and striking, and Symone could picture strangers stopping on the street to stare at her.

Carol had recently separated from her partner, whom she described as abusive, someone who was bad for her and her family and whom she wanted out of her life. She revealed that she had a history of abuse. She was sexually assaulted by other men years before, both times leading to the births of her two older daughters, ages nineteen and twenty-one. "I recently shared with them how they were conceived," she said solemnly.

Symone found herself in familiar territory, almost able to predict Carol's next words. For the past year, Symone had been working at a legal organization that supported people affected by interpersonal violence and domestic abuse. The detached, easy way Carol spoke of these life events struck Symone, and she felt herself responding in kind, dissociating from the words as she nodded along.

"He started telling me, 'This isn't my kid' and 'How can you prove this is even mine?' Things like that. He would totally disappear. Then he would show up with presents or agreeing to pay the rent because he knew I lost my job." So Carol, a former legal secretary who "knew people," decided to look into his background and found a legal case open against him. His former wife was prosecuting him for ripping off his stepdaughter's panties. "They have a restraining order against him . . . It's awful." She paused. "I have an eleven-year-old girl. I just don't feel safe having him around."

Symone tried to catch Erica's eye to no avail; she was engrossed in Carol.

"So this is why I need the two of you. I don't have anyone else otherwise." The fluorescent bulbs were stark next to the darkness of the night, of Carol's words.

"Of course. We are here for you," Erica said.

"Definitely," Symone agreed distractedly, excusing herself to use the bathroom. She needed a break. *Something doesn't feel right*, she said to herself in the cloudy mirror.

For the first time ever, she questioned whether she should take on a birth. "I remember [Carol's story] resonating because at the time I was going through my own breakup and had a lot of associated feelings with that," she says now. "I was feeling really downtrodden. And I was doing [domestic violence] legal work at the time, and so as we spoke, there were lots of click moments . . . and I kind of wrote them off as being part of being this person's doula. But also being tempted to not do the birth because I felt like I was getting it from both ends. I felt really burnt out and miserable doing domestic violence (DV) legal work, and I felt terrible about that, because I wanted to give my all and manage my own personal life."

Initially in her career, Symone had been drawn to domestic violence work, connecting to it through her very first job at a local abortion fund. It was January 2007 when she walked into the open, drafty office, at that time housed in an art gallery in Chelsea, the cataclysmic moment of her activism. At seventeen, she didn't know much about feminism or reproductive rights. She had cold-called a few organizations in the city, a blabbering kid on a phone interview, and the fund had given her a shot.

The falling snow threw a blinding pall against the large gallery windows as she folded herself into a seat among eight other similarly squished workers. Like most first days on the job, she didn't really know what to do or what to expect. She felt let down as she spent the morning checking emails and reading client files, imagining that this was the professional world and her unremarkable destiny. As the day passed, she clicked back to the voice messages she'd already checked multiple times, expecting to hear about a delay in an order of ink cartridges.

Instead, she heard a powerful story that was at once unfathomable and deeply resonant in her consciousness. A clinic advocate had called. *A client was raped crossing the Mexican border, is pregnant, and needs an abortion. Please help.* Symone hadn't realized that the small fund was using the same phone line for vendors and clients. She hastily scribbled down the clinic's information, her heart quickening, and listened to the next message: *A DV survivor from New England has just left an abusive partner, is living in a shelter with her two-year-old, and can't have another baby. She needs an abortion. Can you help?*

Nothing in Symone's life had prepared her for these calls. She knew little about domestic violence or abortion or immigration, but she knew what fear sounded like. She knew that what was tugging at her insides and clicking in her brain and buzzing in her ears wasn't going away. "There was a story attached to these people's lives for the first time," she remembers. "And one that I had never been privy to and was protected from. I never thought about domestic violence as something you had to leave. I never thought about people crossing the border or people who had experiences that were against them or acted upon them."

Suddenly Symone knew that what she was doing mattered. Picking up the phone mattered. Ordering the ink cartridge mattered. Listening to stories mattered.

But that day at the diner, five years later, Symone was feeling far away from that moment at the abortion fund and miles from her activist roots. She wasn't quite sure what was going on within her, but she was tired and unfocused. Warning bells were sounding.

When she got back to the table, Carol said, "I'm the one who's pregnant, and you keep using the bathroom!"

"What? Oh." Symone smiled weakly, not even realizing she had used the bathroom-escape trick once before. As Carol continued to talk, Symone noticed her own hands balled into tight fists—the paper napkin in her lap entirely shredded, seemingly by her own fingers. Each word Carol spoke felt like an explosion in Symone's ears. She wanted to duck under the table.

Instead, she hurriedly collected the pieces of napkin, placing them next to her cup of chamomile tea. She peeked over at Erica who was sitting beside her. Erica remained locked on Carol, her eyes wide with concern. Symone felt confused by her own reaction—she didn't know that this was what the beginnings of burnout looked like. How could she? Often direct-care workers don't know exactly what their breaking point will be or when it will occur. Burnout tends to be something that socks you in the face out of nowhere; you only find its obvious trail after the damage has been delivered and you are picking up your own broken pieces.

Symone made the decision to rejoin Carol and Erica, knowing that despite her misgivings she would take on this client. After all, she was young and had a lot to prove. She didn't say no to things, especially not clients who needed her help. "One big flaw I had as a doula was giving too much of myself," she reflects, a common trait of a passionate high achiever. "I used to do a ridiculous amount of birth shifts, almost in a competitive way, and if shifts were open I would take them. There were times when I was in clinic six times a month. I think there is this person in me that wants to be seen as reliable."

That day, the three women stepped onto the long road of winter together. It felt never-ending as Symone and Erica spent the next three months moving from one extreme to the next with Carol. On top of everything, Carol was a single mom of four, had just lost her job, and was possibly getting evicted. And, of course, Jason wasn't going away easily.

There was the time when Carol emailed them from her bathroom floor, crying because Jason had screamed at her and wouldn't take her to her prenatal appointment. There was the time in late January when they went to her baby shower, a day of celebration poisoned with stories of Jason's evil. Symone, a longtime vegetarian, found herself eating meat in her anxiety, eyeing her smartphone as Carol's nine-year-old son tugged it from her grip to play a game.

But there was also the noticeable love between Carol and her children. They formed a tight unit. Her oldest daughter was helping her take care of the younger kids, all while managing her own relationship and school. Carol often shared how grateful she was for her daughter and how thrilled she was to have her at the birth. As the due date drew closer, Symone clung to the moments of hope, finding herself—to her surprise—almost looking forward to the birth. She was at least ready for it to be over.

That morning in March, when Carol announces that she is in labor, Symone leaves work early for the hospital. Doulas with full-time jobs often struggle to find employers that will allow them to leave work to attend a birth, and Symone is grateful to her agency for giving her that freedom.

On the way, her phone buzzes again. "Jason is here with me. And my daughter isn't going to be able to come. You know, now there isn't enough room."

Symone's first reaction to the chain of events that unfolds that day is anger. She has come to know the realities of DV and the frequency of reunion, and yet the amount of emotional energy she has expended listening to the terrible things this man has done feels wasted.

"Of course we understand," she and Erica assure Carol at the hospital, because doulas don't judge or have feelings about their clients in front of their clients.

Symone has always prided herself on being reasonable, coolheaded, and action oriented. As a doula, she describes herself as nonthreatening: she makes her clients feel immediately safe and at ease. She is quick to laugh, like she either saw the joke coming or simply wants to make you feel comfortable with what you said. She asks for feedback, not because she always needs it—she figured it out long before you came into the picture—but because she wants to include you and foster connection. As a co-doula, she takes the collaboration seriously and professionally. She focuses on creating an egalitarian partnership and often assumes the role of teacher.

Yet this time around, she finds herself letting Erica take a subtle lead, withdrawing ever so slightly so that neither Erica nor Carol really notices. "In some ways I felt [Erica] formed a better relationship with the client. There were some weird dynamics in terms of race," remembers Symone, who is a woman of color. "The client was Jamaican American but talked about Asian family members and Caucasian family members she had—there was an exoticism of this other [Caucasian] doula. But beyond that, Erica had a lot more flexibility than I had. She didn't work full-time and was able to come to midday lunches with this client and be supportive in a way that didn't feel comfortable for me since this client felt like a replication almost of the clients I worked with ten hours a day at my legal job."

Withdrawing from your clients, building an impenetrable fortress around yourself, can often signal burnout. Symone wants to look away from Carol at every turn, as if she is bracing herself for a final, tragic blow. She simultaneously finds herself becoming cynical and detached. "Here we go *again*," she often thinks. And yet—because of the insidious nature of burnout—she cannot see it waving its red flag. She just feels like a bad person and a shitty doula.

Back in the waiting room, Symone's phone beeps and a message from Erica appears: "Carol is getting an epidural." Symone winds her way through the hall to the bank of elevators, texting Erica back, "Coming up." The doors open, and she steps inside, fighting the urge to press all the buttons and ride it to the top and back down again.

She finds Jason and Erica in the labor and delivery waiting room, a closet-sized space allocated for family members. The nurses who guard the room from their station across the hall eye her with an equal mix of boredom and suspicion. Though not thrilled to be back in such close quarters with Jason, Symone finds she can relax in the more serene environment. She studies him. He appears almost faceless to her, distant but hovering—a shadow.

"We've only been here a few minutes," Erica says.

Symone nods and takes a seat. Epidurals can take anywhere from fifteen to forty-five minutes to administer, depending which medical staff are involved and how the patient takes to the drug. Guests are asked to leave the room during this time period.

While birth doulas are typically recruited to assist mothers through drug-free vaginal deliveries, commonly known as "natural births," the Doula Project is often brought in for various other reasons. These include providing general guidance for first-time parents, supporting individuals laboring alone or making adoption plans, and advocating for pregnant teenagers or undocumented people. While many of these folks also prefer an unmedicated vaginal birth, it is not always the first priority.

Symone considers that the epidural might drag the labor out even further, as it is known to do. One school of thought says this happens because its numbing effects slow down the normal functioning of the pelvic floor muscles, which help create contractions that dilate the cervix. Symone quietly mentions this to Erica, who still manages to appear fresh and alert. Symone feels like an ogre next to her, grimy and miserable.

Their conversation is interrupted by the sound of crying and a nurse bursting into the room, "Your son is here!" They race down the hall toward the screaming baby. Jason is leading the way, almost running. Symone feels a pang of sympathy for him. Despite everything, he was excited about the birth.

The nurses meet them at the door of Carol's room with wide smiles, "Oh, you should *all* come in! Can you believe it? She just turned right over, and there he was!" Symone suspects the two-person limit is being overlooked and that the friendliness is being turned up, both out of genuine happiness at seeing a baby born and an understanding that the three of them experienced a loss in missing the birth. As a doula—when supporting a client through a difficult labor—being present for the birth is crucial for your soul and your sense of closure. Birth doulas have a specific end goal and much of it culminates the moment the baby is born. Even though Symone had wanted to avoid the room, she is pained over missing the birth.

Carol greets them weakly, but her eyes are bright. "I felt like I needed to push, right as they were giving me the epidural. I just laid on my side, and he came out!" Carol is forty-two, and this is her fifth birth. The doctors didn't even wait for her to dilate ten centimeters, they just let her push, and he was born a few minutes later, leaving the epidural incomplete. "Symone, look, look at his finger. This means he's special." The baby has an extra finger attached to his pinky.

Jason is at the bed, a cloying arm draped over Carol. Symone feels herself recoil at the gesture, one marked more by possessiveness than affection. She listens uncomfortably to their whispering. "My little boy, my little boy, I'm gonna buy him so many nice things, I'm gonna take care of him."

The postpartum shine misses Symone entirely. She checks the clock continuously and offers canned, rote responses: "Congrats on the baby! I'm here whenever you need me. We should leave the two of you alone. I'll come visit again tomorrow!"

At last she breaks out into the night air and climbs onto the I train, exactly one hour after the delivery. But she still feels uneasy. She senses that even though the birth is over, typically signaling finality for the doula-client relationship, her time with Carol is far from finished.

"Symone! Symone!" Carol's frantic voice comes through the phone the next morning, a jumble of cries and stutters.

"Carol, what happened?" Symone closes her eyes, wincing.

"He took my food and left . . . he's gone! He took my sandwich!" Carol sobs.

Her children had not been able to attend the birth, but they had thoughtfully packed a bag of food for Carol: apple juice, peanut butter and jelly sandwich, snack packs—all of their favorites. When Jason saw the bag, he had yelled and said he wasn't being taken care of, that Carol had the hospital food, and he had nothing. He took her sandwich and disappeared.

"I'm so sorry, Carol. That's awful."

Later in the day, Symone gets another message from Carol, saying there is an emergency and she needs Symone and Erica to come to the hospital to meet with the social worker immediately. Jason had called her room, and she put him on speakerphone so her kids could listen while he berated her. He yelled that this was his child, and he could see him "whenever the fuck he wanted." It has only been thirty-six hours since she gave birth.

Symone squeezes into the room with Carol's friends, all crowded around her offering words of support. "I want Jason banned from the hospital," Carol tells the social worker. "And I want to change all the locks on my door. Babies," she says to her kids over the phone, "whatever you do, don't open the door, okay? Your stepdad is dangerous, and he's gonna hurt the baby. Do you understand?"

Symone tries to shield the horror on her face, pinching at her nose and looking down. Admittedly, she has been to way more physically taxing births than Carol's and has spent days caring for her clients with little food or sleep. But her emotional state has never been twisted up this way before. "Every dynamic triggered me," she remembers. "Every disagreement. Being around folks with tough circumstances, and there is no easy end because these are people's lives. People don't pause for you. And it was not a healthy choice for me to do DV work in tandem with being a doula because I was burning the candle at both ends."

The next morning, a stream of texts comes through her phone. Carol needs to change her locks. Now. Can Symone's legal agency help?

Carol becomes Symone's client again. This time at her full-time job, a boundary she has never crossed before. Symone moves quickly, contacting the locksmith and providing Carol with information about orders of protection and child support. But there are issues. Carol and Jason are legally married and live in public housing, so Jason has the right to enter the apartment. He also has the right to see his baby.

As the week goes on, a gnawing fear gives way to what is so disturbing about this situation: Carol has Symone's personal cell number. None of her legal clients do. They can't call her in the middle of the night saying, "Oh my God, my life is over," or "Why didn't the locksmith come yet, I've been waiting all day."

Symone stays up late worrying, *What if the locksmith doesn't show? What if Jason breaks into the house and does something to the kids? What if he takes the baby?* She feels a crushing in her chest, the sense that she is suffocating. *If something happens to them, it's on me.* Her head begins to spin, a blur of all the survivors she has seen over the past year. Carol's face whirls most prominently, round and round, until, finally, Symone falls into a deep black sleep.

A few days later, she receives the following text from Carol, blandly stating: *"They changed the locks. Thank you."*

She doesn't hear anything else for six months.

Symone is lost in the Bronx.

She stops a stranger on the street, "Excuse me, could you help me find this address?" She points to a scrap of paper she's written on, wiping sweat from her brow with the back of her hand. It's July, four months after Carol's birth, and she's trying to find the apartment of a woman named Annabelle. Annabelle is her new client, her first since Carol.

The stranger shrugs. He doesn't know that street. Symone sighs deeply, frustrated, and wonders if this is a sign.

Maybe she isn't ready to take on a birth yet? But she keeps walking. She had liked Annabelle's voice over the phone and her answers on the online application all potential Doula Project clients are asked to fill out.

When Symone finally reaches her destination, she is buzzed upstairs. Annabelle's apartment grabs her at once, pulling her into a warm, welcoming hug. Plush pillows are scattered over a deep leather couch. Gold-framed mirrors hang on the walls. An astrological guide is taped to the refrigerator. Inspirational quotes line the tabletops. Symone is most struck by a huge poster stating, "This Life Is Yours."

Annabelle pats the couch cushion next to her, and they both sit cross-legged with their shoes off. Symone quickly flashes back to the cold diner she met Carol in last winter.

The dozens of questions Symone prepared never leave her bag. Her pen remains tucked in its side pocket. They talk for hours—about Annabelle's sixteen-year-old daughter, about her infant son who was killed in a car accident years before, and about the love of her life whom she has known since childhood but has only recently begun a relationship with. "I hadn't been with anyone for fourteen years. I told him, 'I don't need you unless you respect me always.' And he has." Symone's heart fills. It has been a while since she has been near a loving relationship.

Left off the Doula Project application is the news that Annabelle is also a DV survivor and will be delivering at West Side Hospital. Symone fleetingly thinks, *What the fuck, universe?* Yet, maybe this is meant to be, maybe this is the birth that will help her heal.

A few weeks later, Symone helps welcome Annabelle's child into the world, surrounded by Annabelle's daughter, partner, and aunt. The hospital room is a replication of Carol's, but this one is filled with sun and love. A photo of Annabelle's deceased son, looking down on her and her newborn, is taped to the wall above her bed. "Symone, do you want to hold him?" Annabelle puts him in Symone's arms. "Honey, get a picture!" she says to her partner.

The nurse walks in. "You know you could be related to them?"

Symone laughs, "I wouldn't mind that!"

She leaves her legal job a month later.

That November she goes to Carol's apartment for lunch. She's had time to understand that much of her experience with Carol reflected a negative place in her own life. She now knows intimately that common self-care trope: *you can't take care of others unless you can take care of yourself.* "When you're in the midst of it," Symone says, "it can feel normal. And then when you're out of it, you're like, that is really fucked up, I can't believe I lived that way."

Today, she is far from her breakup and her legal job, happily working as a freelance doula. She has shared her story of burnout with others as a cautionary tale but also as a means of personal healing, of letting others in to care for her. For Symone, this lunch with Carol is an opportunity to close off an old chapter.

She sits at the kitchen table while Carol prepares the food and catches her up on the children and Jason. She took him back a few times until he humiliated her in the middle of the street in front of her neighbors, calling her a whore. As she speaks, Symone remembers why she left DV: she had begun to think the world was a duplicitous, unsafe place.

Nevertheless, as Carol continues, for the first time Symone does not feel the tightening in her chest. The mood is different from before; Symone is different. And Carol seems happy. She is enamored of her baby, her family. "I just made a decision finally, and I'm committed to raising my kids on my own."

Carol offers Symone a plate, a pescatarian feast made especially for her. She is touched that Carol remembered her diet and went out of her way even though she is still unemployed. Carol joins her at the table, son in her lap. He steals bits of food off her plate. "How's your fish?"

"So delicious, thank you."

"I bought a cranberry cheesecake from Whole Foods, so save some room." They smile across the table at each other.

Symone steps out onto the street, at peace with her decision to see Carol one last time. She reflects:

Being a doula, you can only control for so much. These are just living, vital people, and things change. So even though I wished [Carol] had fit into some mold, things change, and I'm not in the room with her and her partner deciding [on] parenting or being together or any of those things. And I think that being a doula has taught me to be more comfortable with change. It's still tough for me, but

I'm learning to be comfortable with how things evolve or people evolve and that they aren't perfect. There's just so much there that precedes my relationship with them. And it's taught me so much about how to be a person and just let go and figure out this is what I can do, this little tiny piece. And the rest of it I can't carry with me.

Burning Out and Coming Back
Annie and Lila

Annie is back. She bounds through Brooklyn, crossing busy streets jammed with morning commute, dodging the rush of pedestrians trying to get to work on time. Her heavy tote bag beats like a drum against her hip, her long golden-brown hair tangles with the wind as she weaves her way to her destination.

She reaches Planned Parenthood and pauses for a moment to take in the scene, breathing in its familiarity. The simple, unmarked building might be mistaken for any other kind of business if not for the few fair-weather protesters halfheartedly waving signs but mostly drinking coffee and talking to each other. They politely say good morning and offer her a "Jesus Saves" pamphlet as she bounces lightly up the stairs. She tells them, "No, thank you."

It's her first time in months working as a doula, having recently taken a hiatus to address her own crisis of self-care. For a period of time, Annie had completely thrown herself into the Doula Project. She was a site coordinator for Planned Parenthood and sat on the leadership circle, all while balancing a short list of paying jobs that were, at best, less than satisfying. At the same time, she was trying to figure out her next steps after finishing a master's degree in Narrative Medicine, where she and Lauren had met. Everything was tenuous. She thought maybe she would go to divinity school—she even got into one of the top programs—but the reality of it . . . The closer she came to going, the more she realized she was about to plunge into something that she just didn't want to do. She knew she wanted a career where she could take care of people. But how? She looked at a list of unknowns, she considered her dissatisfaction, and she didn't have any answers. It made her terribly sad, terribly stressed. She felt so much doubt in everything and an unbearable, clinging sense of shame for a reason she did not want to articulate, because saying it out loud would make it more real.

Thinner and thinner.

She was familiar with the warning signals of the eating disorder she had struggled with for the past fourteen years. She tried to push them away, ignore them, convince herself that she could keep going by saying, "Oh, no, my eating disorder isn't *that* bad. I'm okay."

But deep down she knew better—she was, in fact, *not* okay. She was scraping the bottom of wellness. The overwhelming feeling of shame that came from dealing with the same issue for so damn long, an issue that still haunts her from her teenage years, was crippling. She knew what she had to do: put everything else in her life down and figure out what she needed to do to survive.

When Annie left the city that summer, she said tacitly that she was dealing with a "chronic medical issue" and promptly checked into a treatment program. She exchanged goodbyes with friends and doulas and left as quickly as she could. She didn't expect to look back.

In social justice circles the term "self-care" can have a polarizing effect on activists and care providers. On the one hand, everyone exalts self-care as necessary, important, and nourishing. "How can you take care of anyone else if you're not taking care of yourself?" we cry.

But others cringe when "self-care" comes up in conversation. A colleague of ours sums it up well: "I hear people begin to talk about self-care, and the only thing I hear is, 'you're about to screw me over by ducking out of something.'"

No matter how much we understand its necessity, self-care can be a source of real tension in activist communities, where it feels like there is so much to do and never enough time or manpower to do it. The conversation gets even more fraught when we turn to doula work, a form of activism through direct care, where our job is physically and emotionally draining and contingent on everyone holding up their end. Canceling a doula shift means that clients go unserved, and any absence on our part works against us in our clinic relationships. Attending a birth means that you are ready to suspend a lot of your usual needs and comforts—a bed, a warm meal, a shower—until the baby is delivered.

For many years at Doula Project trainings, the leadership circle would awkwardly joke about who was the most qualified to run our workshop on self-care.

We would laugh nervously. "Who remembers to sleep well and eat three meals a day? Ha, ha, ha."

There would always be an uncomfortable silence as we randomly selected a person to begrudgingly offer to remind new trainees to stay hydrated. Our original self-care workshop was a half hour tacked on to the end of an intense two-day training focused on abortion. We would run down a basic list: "Drink water! Call us if you need to talk, we're here for you! Oh, and if you feel like you're going to pass out, sit down before you fall." Then we would deliver a hypnobirthing self-love meditation that was passed down from an experienced birth doula trainer, reading its lines in one swooping breath.

But none of this does justice to the work we do or to the importance of doulas bringing their best selves to clients at all times. When Annie joined the Doula Project, she became instrumental in reorganizing our doula training so that it emphasizes a *practice* of self-care: an evolving, careful exercise, not a quick moment here or there. She bristles when she hears self-care reduced to "drink enough water" and "get enough sleep." In reality, self-care is a commitment. She makes this explicit, "It's not something that reaches perfection . . . It's a process that requires a lot of patience and a lot of awareness to do well."

When Annie thinks about self-care, she is looking toward a cultural shift that needs to happen for the sustainability of doula work. At the crux of it is self-awareness. She pushes back against the clichéd narratives of self-care: it's not enough to do yoga and eat well or to want to be indestructible. Annie tries to reframe the self-care narrative to emphasize that every moment in every day we make choices around our needs and that we don't have to make them alone. To Annie, self-care is a communal practice that becomes unnecessarily individuated. She says, "Communities are needed so that we can discuss the different choices that we all make and inspire, bolster, and hold each other accountable to these small gestures that we make contact with all the time."

Most of all she reinvigorates the words that doulas and caregivers know to be true, though we can't be reminded enough:

> Self-care is also not just for *you*. The vitality of you and the way you care for yourself is a responsibility you have toward your community, for your community. I don't mean to say that people should feel bad, or we're criticizing people for not knowing their limitations or not taking care of themselves. *And* at the same time, if you're constantly joining a community where you're offering a tremendous act of service to others, you are offering a different degree of responsibility both for the person you're going to support and for the community around you. Any way that you're situating yourself consciously in a community, in a relationship, or in a partnership, you have a responsibility to care for them and to build trust with them—not to self-sacrifice for them but to self-care for them and for you.

Back at Planned Parenthood, Annie feels rooted in herself for the first time in a long time. She takes in the familiar recovery room, the recliner chairs, the graham crackers and ginger ale. The nurses give her a hug and tell her they are happy she is back. It feels good—really good. *This is what I need to be doing,* she thinks. The apprehension that glimmered in her peripheral vision earlier that morning slips away within minutes.

Annie had been a doula for a long time before joining the Doula Project, but from the get-go, she was drawn to full-spectrum work and the kind of care we were providing. She was particularly thrilled for the opportunity to be with clients during experiences of "ambiguous loss," where emotions run the gamut from mourning to relief to confusion. Having been affected by multiple losses in her own life—combined with her abundant empathy—she was adept at caring for clients whose experiences were not expected to be unilaterally joyful.

After being almost constantly on call as a birth doula for a couple of years, she also realized it was better for her own well-being to be doing shift work with clear start and end times. And she wanted to be a member of a community of doulas. Many doulas in New York City often feel unstable and coltish, especially when they are first starting out. Finding mentorship can be difficult. Prior to the Doula Project, Annie felt like a bit of a drifter, independent in a way that was not nurturing even though she was involved with a few different collectives.

Today she feels a capacity to be present with her clients that is beyond anything she has felt before. She is grounded, confident, and self-knowing, as if she has reached a new depth in her feelings about this work, its importance, and her place as a doula. She is more present with herself in a way that she didn't know was possible, especially after working through her own issues of shame, loss, and trauma. It's not that she couldn't connect with people before; she has always been a great doula. It was intuitive to her to be a caregiver. But this . . . this is different.

When she entered her treatment program that past summer, she was expecting the same routine she had experienced before: the message that the end goal for eating disorders is healthy management and maintenance and that recovery isn't possible. She bristled as she waited to hear the familiar well-meaning lectures about how this will always be a part of her life, and it's just a matter of how she is able to live with her eating disorder in order to make it unobtrusive.

She was surprised when she was told that recovery was absolutely within her reach. It sparked a radical change in her perspective. She reflects, "I think that shifted my ability to speak forthrightly about what my experiences are and what my needs are and claim recovery more vocally and with less shame than I had ever been able to do in the past. I do think we learn the same lessons over and over again, and each time it's a little different. This past time I felt like I really sunk to a different level in terms of what I learned."

It was the first time in her life that she understood that recovery was possible. That joy and confidence is with her in the clinic. She is glowing with a love toward herself and everyone else. She can do this—caring for people is what she is meant to do.

Like many doulas, when Annie first trained as a birth doula during her senior year of college in 2007, she dove into the work hard and fast—she has never been one to do anything halfway. She took on an abundance of clients while she was still in school, working with Inwood House. At the same time, she started working with The Icarus Project, a radical mental health collective that is by and for people "who experience the world in ways that are often diagnosed as mental illness."

For two years, she threw herself into both programs, but it was a lot. She was starting to feel herself fade. She knew, distantly, that this lifestyle would probably not be sustainable for too long, but she was happy to do it in the beginning. There was so much about it all that she loved, so she tried to ignore the looming feeling that she might need to stop—or at least slow down—sometime soon. She was on call for births all the time, glued to her phone, never well rested: someone might need her at any moment.

In the middle of all that, in 2009, Annie answered the phone and learned that her father had taken his own life. And everything—everything—lost its vibrancy in the face of that loss.

She found the ideas of "coping" or "moving on" impossible in the immediate aftermath of her father's death. It was like walking with a broken leg. Looking at the loss straight on was excruciating, so she averted her gaze. She remained on call for her birth clients.

A few weeks after the memorial service she went to what she would later call "the most traumatic birth I've ever done."

She was with a young couple, Johanna and Richard, at one of the nicer hospitals in the city, working with a kind, wonderful labor and delivery nurse who was supportive of this soon to be new family. Annie was hanging on by a string, faking her way through a state of total breakdown. She put on a gentle affect and offered encouraging words, but she felt sick. She knew she shouldn't have there.

The doctor managing the labor was one of the nightmare OBs Annie had heard about but never encountered up until that point. As Johanna was pushing, the doctor screamed at her, frustrated by the complicated labor and probably aware of a looming emergency. The baby was stuck, and it was dangerous. Out of necessity, the doctor had to push hard against Johanna's perineum, the bottom of her vagina, to get the baby out. She screamed as she tore badly under the pressure of the baby's head and the doctor's hands.

Annie held her client tight for comfort, as much for herself as anyone else. Her head was pounding. In one ear she heard the baby crying, the announcement that everything had ended up okay. The nurse brought the baby over to distract Johanna, who was deliriously happy, almost oblivious to—or perhaps, willing to ignore—the violence that Annie had witnessed.

Annie offered a hollow smile. She pushed a strand of hair away from her face and realized it was bloody. She looked down. There was blood everywhere: it covered her shoes, the floor. The doctor and his assistant exchanged tense whispers and hustled between Johanna's legs to repair the tear as she cooed to her new baby.

When Annie got home she collapsed onto the floor of her bathroom and vomited. As she climbed into the hot shower, she questioned everything she had done or not done that may have contributed to this awful birth. Worse, how could she say that the birth was "awful" when her client ended up being so happy? How could she see this client again, and say, "Hey, your birth was one of the most deeply wounding experiences I will ever have, but I'm glad you're doing well?"

It took another few months of pushing it before, on a day in October, Annie fell onto her bed, broken and sobbing, thinking, *I just . . . I can't. I need to stop. I need to stop.*

So she did.

Annie has learned that it's not enough to be invested in doula work politically or even to *want* to do it. Bringing your full self to your clients requires a process of self-care and embracing your own vulnerability to be authentic.

Maybe the difference now, she thinks, is that she has come to own her vulnerability, which is integral to her understanding of self-care. She encourages a practice of accepting vulnerabilities and embracing them, but at the same time, not living in a place of victimhood. She views self-care as parallel to self-awareness and sees the importance of bringing her own humanity to encounters with clients.

She can't help but be "sympathetically frustrated" when activist and caregiving communities are so resistant to real conversation about self-care, because at this point she can't imagine doing this work without it. She acknowledges that a

lot of caregivers and activists resist it because of how externally motivated they often are:

> It's really uncomfortable. The actual work for self-care
> is going into your depths and your weaknesses and your
> vulnerabilities and your proclivities and getting really hon-
> est with yourself—where, actually, activists are inclined to
> look outward. We look to the other and think about what's
> going on. The focus is external a lot of the time. Even if
> it's internal, personal things that have brought them to this
> work in one way or another, I think that activists by and
> large, myself included, have a lot of the time wanted to
> push the spotlight on the other person in order for light to
> not be shined on [themselves]. Because it's uncomfortable!
> And it's humiliating! You're going to face a lot of the stuff
> you've acquired over the course of your lifetime, and that
> is an icky and vulnerable process. I don't know if it's just
> activists, but I think there are particular types of person-
> alities that activists often have in terms of wanting to be
> incredibly caregiving and self-sacrificing and all of this, but
> I think people in general have resistance to doing this kind
> of introspective work because it's some of the hardest stuff
> you can do.

She reflects on all of this in the brief lull before patients start
coming in for the day, until a young woman walks into the
waiting area. She is maybe about eighteen or nineteen years
old, the age when many people are on the cusp of being
independent. Her name is Lila. She is quiet, curious. The
muscle memory of doula work takes hold, and Annie jumps

back into the routine of the clinic—walking Lila back into the procedure room and helping the nurses get her set up for her abortion.

Lila is remarkably calm about the procedure, neither deeply distressed nor apparently numb. She locks her gaze on Annie's hazel eyes and asks her the question that almost all doulas hear at least once: "Have you ever done this before?"

"No, I haven't. But I have taken care of many people who have, and I will be by your side as much as you need or want me to be."

Lila squeezes Annie's hand. They remain entwined throughout the procedure.

Twenty minutes later and now in a postabortion haze of medication, Lila sips her ginger ale in the recovery room and asks Annie a series of existential questions: "Who is this guy I'm with?" "Do I let my mother make too many of my decisions?" "What do I want?"

Annie responds gently and coaxes Lila to think through it all a little more by asking her questions. Tears stream down Lila's face, but she is not bothered. Even crying seems appropriate, matter-of-fact, honored as an important part of the process by Lila. Annie is struck by it—how it almost seems like she has already had a life of profound self-awareness that most people can't even begin to imagine. She feels like she and Lila are mirrors for one another, offering support and eye contact, holding hands, exposing the unconditional love between strangers that arises in doula care.

There is an exchange of questions: Lila wants to know about Annie, what she thinks and why she is here to take care of people having abortions since she hasn't had an abortion herself. Her questions aren't hostile—just inquisitive. Annie answers anything Lila wants, even some of the details about herself, like her eating disorder, that might have unnerved her before. But now, she's okay with showing her clients her rawness—she is okay with knowing she does not have answers but instead has processes. She says:

> I'm by no means wrapped up in a little package of things I've figured out, but something that helps me when I get in that [emotional place with a client] is allowing myself to be with someone else and taking the deep breaths, talking it out, whatever it may be. . . . If someone is swirling in their head, as sometimes happens, I say, "Let me be your anchor, hold my hand, let's breathe together." We're coming in together.

Annie understands that being aware of personal vulnerability redirects hierarchy in caregiving: it's not about the doula protecting the client but rather a dynamic of humility, where the doula leaves space for the client to direct her own healthcare. She says:

> The idea [as a doula] is that you've done the work around this stuff, you can bring it in as your experience, and you don't need to be holier than thou. You can say, "This is stuff I deal with on a daily basis." Anything I offer as a doula is often based out of my experience—what I've seen work for others too, but very much what I've seen that's worked for myself. If you are attuned with yourself, and

you present that, you're going to be a more trustworthy companion for your client. If you're showing up with your vulnerabilities, if you're showing up with an authenticity to the way that you're speaking about the tools you're offering, it generates trust in a way that's different than something didactic and authoritarian.

It's time for Lila to leave so the small clinic can make room for the next patient. There is nothing left to do, so she and Annie hug, holding each other so, so tightly before Lila walks away.

How to Self-Care

A mini chapter in which we share some of our favorite self-care techniques.

You Can't Take Care of Anyone Else Unless You Take Care of Yourself

Okay. So we know that a core tenet of doula work is that it's not about you. It's not. You're there to be a supportive, loving, *completely selfless* presence, right?

But *you can't take care of anyone else unless you take care of yourself.* That statement has been dulled into a platitude in a lot of communities, but that doesn't make it any less true. Full-spectrum doula work is amazingly fulfilling, but it can be really *hard.* Sometimes you will not like something your client does or says. Sometimes you will realize that you've run from supporting a birth to supporting abortions all day and you haven't eaten. Most days are beautiful, and you can see a bright light in the work you're doing. Other days you may walk away angry, stressed, or fried.

You are not Florence Nightingale (unless you are, in

which case, we'd like your autograph). You do not need to be perfect. You are allowed to have strong feelings about the work you're doing, and you're allowed to feel like you need to step back. You're only human. No one expects you to be anything else.

Do Not Be a Martyr

By shouldering your clients' burdens you are not taking them away. If your client can't eat during labor, that doesn't mean you should starve in solidarity. It doesn't mean that you should let a client dig their nails into your hand enough to draw blood—a thousand times no. No amount of suffering on your end will relieve suffering for your client. No one wants you to be a martyr, especially not your clients: martyrdom does *not* make you a better doula. Poonam Dreyfus-Pai emphasizes:

> Doula work is not about martyrdom—it's about showing up fully and authentically for someone during a major life transition. If you are not in a place to do that, for whatever reason, that's okay—let someone else do it. Schedule yourself for a reasonable amount of shifts, take breaks from time to time, and have a supportive buddy or team to debrief with when you're done. Get good sleep before a shift, *breathe* throughout, and sit down from time to time. Cry when you're done, or laugh—whatever feels like a release. I made a little ritual for myself where I would have a burger from In-N-Out after my doula shifts in Santa Rosa. It felt so nice to indulge after some hard work.

Time Management and Boundaries:
Be Honest, Be Trustworthy

As a doula your ceiling of tolerance for how much work you can take on will likely become high. So will your ability to stay awake for hours on end and to sleep folded over yourself in a chair or on the floor. If you are working as part of a full-spectrum doula group, remember that your colleagues are depending on you. This work can't happen without a group effort.

That said, in our experience the worst thing you can do is overestimate the amount of time you are willing or able to give. Not only will you find that you burnout fast, but also when it happens you may realize that it is urgent. Without advance notice the program you are in might be hurt by your unexpected absence. The people you work with need to trust you and your ability to be honest about what you can commit to at any given time. It is almost always better to be a little too conservative about your time than to wring yourself dry.

Let Go of What You Can't Control

You're not responsible for the place that your client has chosen to give birth or have her abortion. You have better ways to spend your energy than stressing about whether or not you should have convinced her to go with a different practice that has a lower C-section rate. You are not responsible for her C-section. You are not responsible if she went through with an abortion she ultimately didn't really want to have.

You are there to be a witness, to serve as a guide when necessary, and to validate your client by letting her know that you see her and you care about her story. That doesn't mean you can change it—nor does it mean that she wants you to.

Find a Mentor

We have learned that talking regularly to another full-spectrum doula can be the best form of self-care. We hear and witness things we need to release, things that we can't hold in. Sharing with another like-minded colleague can be healing.

Kat Broadway, abortion doula, says, "Find a doula that is senior to you that you trust. Someone [to whom] you can say, 'This is crazy, I'm really upset about this, this doctor said something fucked up and I don't know what to do,' or 'This client said something fucked up and I don't know what to say.' Empathy and acknowledgment is the best self-care, that is the kind of self-care we can allow ourselves safely."

Guided Meditations, Y'all

Or yoga. Or aromatherapy. Or cooking. That self-love meditation from the Hypnobirthing Institute we mentioned earlier. Whatever. Do something quiet to decompress, something that can help you process the day you've had. And yes, we know that this advice is reinforcing all kinds of doula stereotypes, and we're okay with that.

Burnout Is Real and It Is Sneaky: Check In with Yourself

Janna Slack, founder of the LA Doula Project, says:

I'd heard about it, and I knew it was possible, but I didn't grasp the magnitude of the havoc burnout could wreak in my life—the damage I would sustain to my mental and physical health. There were other things going on that contributed to my burnout, including a move to another state, but as an anxiety-prone person, I hadn't really considered how being on call for three to five births each month might affect me. If you aren't checking in with yourself regularly, it can sneak up on you, and for me, it's taken years to recover from. It's not like the movies where you can go on a girls' trip to Mexico for a week and make it all better.

When I first got into doula work, I thought I had to do everything immediately, right now, yesterday—start a doula project, attend five paying births each month, be involved in activism, serve on the board of my doula association, plan fundraisers. Life is a marathon, not a sprint. You have time to get to all the things you want to do, and they will be sweeter rewards if you are able to enjoy them in the fullness of your mind, body and spirit.

I fell into the Superwoman trap, trying to be all things to all people, not knowing how to find support for myself, or let others help me. I ran on adrenaline for almost a year before the inevitable crash. Please, check in with yourself often and honestly assess what your personal constitution can take. Work with a therapist or coach or mentor who can help you develop sustainable workflow and be honest about what you're able to take on. Make a priority of exploring, setting and enforcing boundaries, developing an on-call/off-call rhythm that is beneficial in your life, and most of all, paying attention to your physical and mental health.

Care for the Caregiver

As caregivers, it is important we let others take care of us as well. While we are pros at caring for others, we tend to be the worst at allowing anyone else to see us in our own vulnerable moments. There is power in caring for others. When we let another care for us, it can feel as if we are giving over that power, exposing ourselves when we are bruised and downtrodden. But we have found that giving ourselves over to another can be empowering and, above all, healing.

Part 5

Activist Practice

The Deep End
Talia and Danika

Sometimes it is the most basic empathetic impulses that elicit the most major life shifts. A lot of people are drawn to direct care by an unnameable, deep instinct to help other people. Often it isn't any one specific moment that inspires people to say, "I went through a traumatic event, and now I want to dedicate my life to fighting back against that," or "I had a personal experience, so I can relate to what a patient might be going through." When we speak to doulas and providers alike—or even when people ask us why we do what we do—it's hard to pin down a general answer. Caregivers may say something like, "Because it's important. I don't know . . . This is something I'm drawn to. It's always been this way." Regardless of why we came to this work, we are here, and we hold a lot.

Doulas in particular are adept at shouldering a lot of the emotional burden of procedures and births. Many who come to the Doula Project are doing it as part of a larger plan to become medical providers, and they know that doula training will make them better at their job. We have also met countless doulas who have been inspired to become doctors and midwives after spending time in clinics with their abortion and birth clients.

We owe a lot to the providers we work with. The work they do is *hard*. Part of what we try to do as doulas is create a community of support within the medical spaces where we practice. We are lucky to have become close to some exceptional doctors and midwives, many of whom are young and share our activist spirit. They do what they do because they want to create change for the better, and because they care about women. And, like the doulas, their work changes them in ways that are heartbreaking, powerful, and unanticipated.

Some of Dr. Talia Williams's earliest memories include being a Girl Scout, choosing the family cat, going to church camp—and learning about public health from the women in her family. Her mother was a health educator in the mostly African American working-class DC Metro area community where her family lived at the height of the HIV/AIDS epidemic. Talia's mother would bring Talia and her sister along with her as she did outreach and organized events. She brought them with her mostly because she wanted them to be involved, but also because as a single mother, money was hard to come by and babysitters were a luxury. At the age of eight, Talia absorbed information like a sponge. She was fascinated by medicine. She knew more about HIV/AIDS than a lot of adults.

At twelve years old, she announced that not only would she be a doctor, but she was definitely going to become an ob-gyn. Around that time, Talia was staying with her great aunt in Syracuse, New York during a summer break. Her great aunt raised an eyebrow. "Oh?" she said. "Why an ob-gyn, specifically?"

"Because delivering babies is sooo cool!"

Her great aunt nodded. A few weeks later, the two were at what looked like a big picnic to Talia, with lots of people with lots of posters at long tables. Her great aunt walked her over to the Planned Parenthood table and greeted several friends warmly. She introduced them to Talia and then bent down to her. "When you grow up are you going to be an abortion provider? That's what ob-gyns do, too, besides delivering babies."

Talia didn't think twice about it at the time. She nodded, "Sure, if that's what ob-gyns do, then that's what I'm going to do too." It was only years later that Talia realized how radical her great aunt had been.

Flash-forward more than fifteen years: Talia is a fellow of the Reproductive Choices Service at City Hospital. Later, she will be promoted to assistant director of the service, and she will specialize mostly in contraception, medical abortion, and obstetrical care. As a fellow, she works closely under Dr. A, director of the service, a respected attending physician who suffers neither fools nor awkwardness lightly.

Dr. A herself came to be an abortion provider somewhat at random, but something compelled her to do it. Her parents balked at first—shootings had just happened at a Boston clinic. And they also reminded her that abortion doesn't necessarily gel with her family's religious Hindu beliefs. But she told her parents that she had accepted a fellowship in reproductive family planning because it meant she could do a master's in public health for free and that a significant amount of money would be put toward her medical school loans. Sure, she was on board with the cause, otherwise why do it? She felt strongly that people should be able to determine their own reproductive lives. But she is also very much a surgeon, and abortion procedures are not exceptionally "surgical." Doing them all day, every day can feel a little redundant, maybe even a little boring, from a medical perspective (though this is not the case from a social or narrative perspective). Still, the fellowship was worth it for Dr. A because she saw the potential to help people, to learn a new surgical skill, and to advance research that is humanistic and patient focused. Practically, doing the fellowship made sense. But there was also something she couldn't quite put a finger on that made her do it, even when she had mixed feelings about abortion becoming such a featured part of her career.

Dr. A will play a primary role in guiding Talia through the sharp learning curve of this unique subset of reproductive healthcare—where patients are socially and medically diverse—and, ultimately, in shaping Talia's practice. Talia comes from a busy but rural hospital in Pennsylvania, where she was never given the option to learn to perform abortions on a regular basis, let alone second trimester procedures. She had a handful of opportunities to do them but certainly not enough to incorporate them into her practice regularly. And yet, that goal she set at twelve years old—"That's what ob-gyns do, so that's what I'm going to do"—turned into a calling. Talia knew that reproductive family planning was what she wanted to do in life. When people ask her "why" she can only think of the strong women in her family who told her this was important.

She learns the ropes of City Hospital. She describes it as "alive. It's like a beast, it's like a living beast." Her days are chaotic and always different. The week begins with a long list of patients who are scheduled for a "booking consultation" where they will get an ultrasound, a gynecological exam, blood work, paperwork, and counseling about what to expect during their procedures. For many patients this is their first visit in years, because they lack health insurance, money, or American citizenship, and are afraid to come in. Talia speaks to people who want anything from contraception to genetic testing to medical or surgical abortion—from anywhere between five and twenty-four weeks. She learns to perform manual vacuum aspiration procedures, laminaria insertions, and D and Es for the first time. She teaches residents and medical students as soon as she has found her own footing.

In doing this fellowship, she opts to defer the authority of being an attending physician for two more years. She finds she is still in a professional place that can be summed up by Britney Spears: "not a girl, not yet a woman." Sometimes it feels like she is back in the space of residency, a little bumbling, confused by the hospital system, and not yet established enough at City Hospital to assert her authority. She is good-natured about it. Clinic coordinators

Melissa and Lauren follow her around with to-do lists and reminders. She is glad that there are doulas to help during the procedures so that she is able to focus on doing a good job (even though she has a good handle on small talk, which is not something that can be said for all providers).

Talia thinks about things holistically in terms of story-based care:

> You hear many stories. "I just had a baby last year" or "my partner died" or "my partner beats me." A lot of it is outside of the procedure, what's going on with the woman and her situation, which had a lot of impact on me saying, "This is the right thing for me; this is exactly what I want to be doing." In terms of the providing, so frequently there, I don't want to say it's routine because it definitely isn't. There were patients for whom the procedure was straightforward, and there were patients for whom it wasn't straightforward, where it was difficult technically, difficult emotionally.

Though Talia sees a wide variety of patients and performs tons of procedures, the ones that stick with her the most are, unsurprisingly, the ones that are the most complicated. During her first month of the fellowship, there is a slew of especially harrowing scenarios: two people have a condition called "placenta accreta," where the blood vessels of the placenta grow into and embed in the tissue of the uterus, "like a flower grows roots in the ground" as Dr. A describes it. This used to be very rare. Now, with the abundance of cesarean births, more and more women are diagnosed, and Talia sees patient after patient who might be at risk for an accreta. But the two patients she sees within the first few weeks of her fellowship have accretas that are especially severe, and she knows their procedures are going to result in hysterectomies. It's bad enough to have to break the bad news to one patient, let alone two. Never mind how nerve-racking it can be to do such complicated procedures. She doesn't think she will ever really get used to it.

She sees teenage patients who are unable to tell their parents they are pregnant. Over and over, in many different languages, she speaks to people who want to talk to her about the children they already have. They show her pictures, and they thank her for her time and her care.

Every week City Hospital's operating room schedule fills up with patients, and every week Talia presides over the procedures. It is hard to anticipate how one might feel before *seeing* a D and E procedure, let alone performing one. They are so fraught within the wider conversation of policy, legality, and morality that navigating the gray areas of emotion as a provider can be tricky.

Some providers are able to compartmentalize better than others. One of the City Hospital attending physicians performed D and Es throughout her own two pregnancies. She did it for the patients who needed the care, and she followed through lovingly and with a smile on her face. But when she was asked about it later, she described the experience as "awful. Just completely awful." She cared about the patients and respected their decisions about their own pregnancies, but that didn't make it easy.

Talia has found her own means to be grounded as she cares for her patients:

> It's part of knowing that you can do something and it immediately has an effect on that person who had the procedure. It immediately positively impacts their life, improves their situations. There is instant gratification. That makes me feel really good. Because I know the weight of it from getting to know them, it makes me feel good in terms of helping to take away this huge burden or situation or heavy thing that someone is dealing with. I think people are often supposed to say it's gruesome, or it's gross, or it's bloody. But I'm not often grossed out or horrified. In general, I feel like when I'm doing a D and E, I'm very focused on the technical aspect and keeping the woman safe. I think that's how I am able to manage it well. In my mind is, *This could be saving her life, this is what she needs, and I want to just keep her safe.* It's more like I feel sometimes more . . . like I'm sorry that it wasn't less messy, for example. I want it to be neat; I want it be done quickly; I want it to be done with respect to the woman and with respect, personally, to me, to the fetus.

It is with humility that Talia reveals what grounds her: her Christian faith. It is something that she often shares with clients, and it deepens her relationship with them. Melissa has found the same—that a spiritual kinship means a special bond and understanding. Their religious beliefs have compelled them to help others in their time of need, to be compassionate and caring when no one else will, and to fill moments of hardship with grace. For many of our clients, their relationship to God is what gives them solace and strength.

The question of religion is one that many of the doulas in the Doula Project struggle with for the simple reason that while many have a relationship with spirituality in some sense, they usually don't identify with a formal or specific religion. Clients will frequently ask doulas and providers questions like, "Do you think God hates me?" or "Do you think I'm going to go to hell?" It can be hard to answer with authenticity and, at the same time, be respectful of a patient's views if you don't share them—particularly when many religions regard women as second-class citizens and abortion as murder.

It is a sad irony that religion and reproductive justice often stand in opposition to one another, especially when we remember that the roots of abortion access before *Roe v. Wade* were in churches. Churches such as the historic Judson Memorial Church in New York—which initiated the Clergy Consultation Service—put women in touch with reputable doctors so that they would be able to have safe procedures. The clergy who participated viewed their work as in alignment with their religious vows and obligations. The whole reproductive justice movement was built on the shoulders of people who were willing and able to channel their religious—often Christian—beliefs into offering love and support to people in a time of need. Now, organizations such as the Religious Coalition for Reproductive Choice are doing a lot of work around ensuring that communities of faith are still part of the support system for doctors, clinics, and patients.

Talia acknowledges the difficulty in balancing her two gut-instincts—one that leads her to God and another that leads her to her calling as an abortion provider:

> Religion is very organized. There are rules, things you're supposed to do, things you're not supposed to do. And abortion is apparently one of those things [you're not supposed to do]. Whatever the situation I recognize that there's a higher power. There's God who made this creature here. I also feel very deeply in some way that this is the path I'm supposed to be on, and this is given to me. This is the road set before me by my higher power. So how can it be wrong?

She acknowledges that those who are religious—including some of the people she sees in church—might push back against that. "They would say that's the Devil speaking," she sighs. "In my heart of hearts I still feel like this is what I want and need to do. Do I feel guilty that I'm breaking some sort of law? Maybe."

Talia has dedicated her whole young life to taking care of other people and still struggles with her calling:

> When I'm at church services, I think about work. I offer up prayers for the families, the patients, the work we do. I ask God to forgive everything that I did that was wrong. And if providing is wrong, well, I do it to help other

people. I think God will understand. It's something I'll struggle with forever, but it's not a bad struggle.

Like Talia, midwife Danika Severino Wynn was drawn to caregiving instinctively. There was no one specific catalyzing moment where she knew that *this* was it. It was more that taking care of people, or, as she would describe it, being a "mothering" type, was integral to her personality. She didn't realize how much this was the case until shortly after graduating from college, when she landed her first nonprofit desk job in development. Her mothering heart beating out of her chest, she intended to be a lawyer so she could advocate for people who needed help. She saw working at a nonprofit as potentially good work experience to take her to that next level. The result? "I wanted to poke my eyes out with a pencil," she says.

Her first experience doing direct care was in college when she worked as an escort and abortion counselor at Planned Parenthood. That was when she got the bug to consider direct care as a potential career. She remarks that her path to becoming a midwife began through her work as an abortion counselor, which in turn fed her fascination with pregnancy, healthcare, and working with people as they began their shift into a new identity as parents. She does not remember when exactly she heard the word "doula," but she knows she was excited that she could work with mothers and babies without having to be a doctor. *This*, she thought, *is what I need to be doing.*

After she attended her first birth as a doula, she was

hooked. It was everything she had hoped for, beautiful and exhausting. She knew for sure that she needed a job where she could interact with and care for people, where she could see she was making a difference. She didn't want to do anything else, didn't want to waste her time pretending she found purpose in her desk job. After a sleepless night she walked into her office and quit.

In retrospect, she is in awe of how lucky she was to have figured out her calling at such a young age. Danika is now a certified nurse midwife (CNM). In order to become a midwife through a CNM program, Danika had to spend time as a nurse for a while and work multiple jobs. She worked as a labor and delivery nurse in two posh New York City hospitals. She also served as a postpartum doula for mothers who had C-sections, and taught childbirth education classes.

Now Danika works at a community-based hospital in a suburb of Providence, Rhode Island. It's basic, no frills. Sometimes it feels like the hospital and the patients are on a small boat in a rough ocean, forced to be sufficient unto themselves without many external resources. She is proud of her work there, proud that the hospital has been able to do so much in the community with so little, and proud that the administration prioritizes her ability to care for her patients consistently. There's a lot that she's able to do there that she wouldn't be able to do anywhere else. She is able to offer compassionate care to patients who are often very marginalized and therefore have limited options. It's important to Danika to be a provider for communities that need it, who wouldn't be able to access this quality of care otherwise. Danika herself grew up nearby, Dominican in a mostly white rural area. She feels a connection here.

Her hospital is similar to City Hospital insofar as what she does every day changes with the demands of the patients. As a midwife, she has the skill to work with people who need gynecological care in addition to those giving birth. On a given day, she might be doing anything from contraceptive counseling for teenagers to changing pessaries for older women suffering from urinary incontinence. She sees patients who need high-risk OB care in consultation with a doctor. This is interspersed with being called back to the labor floor where she can work with her own patients. She can even be the "first assist" at a C-section, which is something that requires extra training but is certainly in the scope of midwifery practice. Being the first assist means that she works closely with the attending surgeon as "the other set of hands in the OR." Mostly it means that if her patient needs to have a cesarean delivery, Danika will still have a major role in her care—she will not have to hand a patient with whom she has developed a trusting relationship over to a doctor that the patient doesn't know.

But unlike any New York City-based hospital or clinic, her hospital is located in what she calls "a health desert." It's in a suburb outside of Providence with public transportation that is so bad that asking someone to get to the city is like "asking them to go to Guam." Patients seeking abortions, which aren't offered at the hospital, or patients who need specialized high-risk OB care often fall through the cracks. She hears many disclosures of abuse and rape. "It's amazing how many people report it when you ask," she says.

She describes a major lack of health literacy in the community and remarks on the contrast to New York. Danika did her initial training in central Brooklyn, an area that has the highest level of maternal mortality in the country. But if people needed help there, she could get them assistance. In addition, the baseline level of knowledge is higher in Brooklyn because there are ubiquitous resources, in the form of clinics, Medicaid laws, and public health initiatives on billboards or ads on the subway.

Danika often finds her patients in Rhode Island overwhelmed with issues and roadblocks. Vulnerable and with few external or public resources—alongside a litany of personal traumas—many are at risk of losing their children to Child Protective Services. After attending patients' births for hours, Danika says, "Seeing mothers go home without their babies is heartbreaking."

She prides herself on being able to keep her work life safely tucked away, compartmentalized from her home life. She focuses on her family: her husband, two young daughters, one a newborn. She spends time lovingly serving as board cochair of the Doula Project. She has a vast network of friends all over the country that she visits as much as she can. But providers often find that their patients live somewhere in the backs of their minds—like the woman Danika saw recently who had been left at the side of a highway by her mother as a toddler and had to have multiple surgeries before the age of four. As an adult, she was now homeless, had just given birth, and was in love with her baby. Sadly, she was declared an "unfit mother" and was separated from her child.

Each night Danika goes home and gets her own daughter ready for bed. She gently lowers her into the bathtub, then pulls on her pajamas afterward. Her daughter alternately giggles and fusses, a happy three-year-old. Some days Danika feels impossibly lucky. Others, she is filled with these stories that follow her wherever she goes.

In particular, Danika recalls her time as a labor and delivery nurse. This is where she "came of age" as a care provider and where she found herself subordinate to the decisions of the doctors and midwives—which proved to be the crystallizing experience in her career. Nurses bear witness to a lot and, like doulas, are limited in their authority to push back against the doctor or midwife who is managing the patient's care. In labor and delivery, Danika found a tenuous and often painful balance of caregiving: most providers—including doulas—choose their profession because they have a drive to ease suffering and want to do it tangibly. And yet, most also find that experiencing trauma on behalf of the patients comes with the territory.

Danika reflects that she experienced the most provider trauma in her role as a labor and delivery nurse rather than as a midwife. There was a list of violations in which she felt implicated: A doctor performed an episiotomy (a surgical cut in the perineum to hasten birth) on a patient who was just beginning to push—who up until that point was laboring without any medical intervention—and then *lied* about it when the patient asked, distressed. There was an emergency C-section that began in a rush before anyone could have been certain the anesthesia took effect. Danika also witnessed anger toward patients who were attempting epidural-free labors, and doctors allowing their own stress to seep out onto the patients. Her job in those moments was to assist, not to meddle—and certainly anyone on the labor and delivery floor would be quick to point that out.

Besides, she says, "When you speak up, you're casting doubt in the patient's mind." But sometimes you can't default to assuming the provider's good intentions are enough when the situation is egregious. After reporting the doctor who performed the episiotomy and then denied it "as she was holding the scissors in her hand," Danika was asked by her supervisor, "And what could *you* have done better in this situation to be more supportive to the doctor?"

And yet, things like episiotomies happen on labor and delivery in the heat of the moment all the time without patient consent—something that rarely happens in any other part of a hospital. The "why" remains confusing. Once, Danika was witness to a particularly disturbing interaction in which a doctor was extremely frustrated by a patient who was insisting on a natural labor to what he felt was her own detriment. It began when the patient came in with signs of a brewing infection after her water had been broken for a significantly long time and ended with some really rough pushing. Danika and one of the other nurses went to check on the patient who told them she was "grateful" to the doctor.

Remembering all of the details of how forceful the doctor was physically and verbally, and how upset the patient was at the end of the labor, Danika felt nauseous.

"When things are really traumatic and really scary, no matter what happens, patients will say, 'Thank you for saving me and my baby.' They just don't know sometimes; they just don't know what's happening [at] the other end of the bed." It was at that point that Danika thought, *Am I putting all my expectations of birth on somebody else? Whose battle am I fighting?*

It's important to emphasize here that there are many wonderful obstetricians, just as there are many wonderful midwives. But as Danika says, caregiving during birth is "innate in some people more than others. And midwives and doctors are all different kinds of people." It's necessary to think about how people in the more subordinate roles within a medical system often get caught between having no decision-making power and holding most of the emotional burden in the room. It is the reality of bearing witness to many different kinds of provider styles during birth. Doulas know this agony well, though in the confines of our role we explicitly opt out of asserting medical expertise. We see a lot. Some of it is incredible, and some of it is horrific. Either way, feeling your own powerlessness in a moment of crisis is painful. Caregiver trauma might be inevitable. Danika says, "It's a field where amazingly beautiful things happen, or amazingly horrifying things happen—traumas of losing a patient or seeing a patient hemorrhage. This is real."

Though challenging for her, Danika says that being a labor and delivery nurse was crucial to her ability to practice as a midwife. There is something to be said about the gratitude one might feel being the decision maker in the room after spending so much time in a subordinate role. Every bad outcome you see, hear, or experience molds your practice. Trauma can be the catalyst that creates provider style. Danika reflects that the process of "unburdening these stories to move forward without all of these bricks on your shoulders" is both profoundly difficult and vital. Otherwise, it becomes who you are as a provider. Danika thinks about the providers she worked with during her time as a labor and delivery nurse. So many of them were so hardened, so calcified by their trauma that they had no faith in the birth process. The trouble is, Danika says, "Birth is not to be feared—it's to be respected. Part of what midwifery means is just being a protector. A crossing guard for birth." She sighs. "If you are so traumatized that you aren't able to go back to that then . . . I don't know. It might be time to get out of the field."

Now that Danika is the primary medical provider in her practice, she is able to curate the decisions in the labor room alongside her patient. She is able to shape the birthing space in a way that will make her patients happy, or at least as happy as possible. Often, she goes back to her doula training as a guiding light for how she practices as a midwife during the "otherworldly aspect of labor." She thinks of the hallmarks of being a doula: holding space, empowering somebody to think of what they can do and what their body can do, and how "human touch can work in a really powerful way."

She also works with a team of doctors she respects immensely. She admits, "I'm sure I'll have some trauma from my own decisions," though given all of her experience as a nurse, she hopes that knowing her decisions were made with good intentions and strong knowledge will soften the blow. And she acknowledges that most people probably feel that way when they become the authority in the room.

Mary jokes that it's the kind of job that *Lifetime* makes movies about. Danika readily admits that, in most ways, she has the "best job in the world." Like Talia, she sees the bright light in her work as a provider, despite the dark turns it sometimes takes. Her patients—and honestly, women in general—are beloved to her. "I feel more and more lucky with what I do, where my life is. Even if I don't like it every day, I love it every day."

She breathes deeply with enormous gratitude.

An Unnameable Place
Kale and Vicki

Kale rushes out of the City Hospital procedure room to catch his train to work. He is one of four original doulas, besides Lauren and Mary, who made it into the clinic that first year.

Kale is not local to New York City—he commutes in from Connecticut, where he works at a neuroscience lab and is getting ready for his move down to Nashville, Tennessee, to pursue his own doctoral study. Later, once he is settled, he will become the founding director of the innovative Trans Buddy program at Vanderbilt University Medical Center. Trans Buddy is an organization that pairs trans people with trained peer advocates, not unlike doulas. This happens after Kale spends two years being professionally plastered to books but personally called upon (by the trans community in Nashville) for help. People ask Kale to come to their appointments and their emergency room visits; they ask him for advice. He is told daily that he is a "safe person."

In 2008 the direct-care bug begins to take hold of him.

Doula work speaks to Kale's experience of spending his entire adult life working in reproductive and social justice. It means a lot to him, though he isn't expecting to be so beautifully winded by it. Being an abortion doula is a little idiosyncratic with his current job at the MRI lab. Luckily, his lab offers him some flexible time, so he comes every Wednesday morning to support clients having first trimester procedures.

He has never done anything like this before. He has no idea, really, what "this" is or if he'll be good at it until he is in the procedure room. He did the training to support the program Lauren and Mary were creating, and because he respected a number of activists who were talking about abortion doulas. Being a birth doula was expensive and time-consuming and maybe not even his thing. Abortion clinic work seemed like a good way to get started. Plus, he and Lauren are friends, and she insisted he join. Kale emanates "caregiver" from a mile away. It makes sense that he would become a doula. He is so often called upon to give general guidance and to help people during times of confusion and grief that he might as well make it a formal role.

Kale and Lauren have known each other since college, where Kale embodied an affect that was both edgy and soft. He is a "loving fighter" who holds you accountable with an unerring compassion. Way back when, Kale had a penchant for ripped punk rock T-shirts, hair dye—particularly on the orange spectrum—and passionately intense conversations. His activism runs through him like blood. He has little tolerance for people who can't wrap their heads around intersectionality. Prior to doula work, Kale had been rooted in doing abortion clinic defense in Cleveland, Ohio, providing medical student education, and generally being invested in social justice at large. But he found that these experiences had not necessarily prepared him for his role in the clinic, where he works by an apparatus of intuition.

Kale runs onto his train with a tenuously held cup of soup in one hand and sighs into his seat, getting comfortable. There's a lot he could do on this train ride. There is always work. He has his books. But his mind is buzzing; he can't think of much besides the morning in the clinic. The weekly train ride is his ritual where he allows himself time to reflect. He closes his eyes as the train moves through the tunnel at Grand Central Terminal and then, poetically enough, rushes into a bright burst of light.

There is a client stuck in his head today, although maybe that's a useless statement because there is a client stuck in his head every day he works as a doula. Mostly he thinks of them after their procedures, which feels like an eternity from when he meets them initially in the waiting room—where so many look frightened, crumpled over themselves. When it's all done they have time to talk. It's so intimate, all of it. They show him pictures of their families; mostly they talk about how great their kids are. He wasn't expecting that his clients would want to talk about their children so much. Often they ask him about God, and he has learned to gently reflect questions back that might help them think through some of what they're struggling with spiritually.

Sometimes he will think back to the day's misgenderings:

at this point in his life, he reads to most people as an androgynous woman. On his first day he didn't think it was necessary to get into the conversation about his gender identity during someone's abortion, so he dressed in his "professional woman costume," wearing khakis and high heels. When he is holding space for someone, he is not thinking about whether or not they are using the right pronoun—something that is important to him in most aspects of his life—he's not really thinking about himself. That doesn't mean it feels great, though. He shifts in his seat.

Today was challenging and strange. He mentally traces his steps through the clinic as he meets Ren, a client who projected a lot of her anxiety about the procedure as pain. Kale tried to be as calm and as soothing as possible, but it was hard to reach her. First, she screamed with all of the air in her lungs as her IV was put in, saying that it was incredibly painful. Kale realized that it's not that it wasn't painful to her—some people *really* don't like needles—but that her feelings of anxiety about the abortion may have made the pain feel even more frightening. She was resigned to the decision in that she was showing up for the procedure. Otherwise, she didn't really have a "choice" as such. She was putting one foot in front of the other. It didn't help that for this procedure she wouldn't be completely asleep. It would just be the medication that amounts to a cocktail in an IV. Most patients do well enough with that, but there are no guarantees.

Ren was uncomfortable throughout the procedure, but when the doctor was more than halfway done she panicked, yelling that it hurt too much, that she couldn't keep going. She pressed her feet into the footrests on the exam table and catapulted back. She started screaming, "I change my mind!" and thrashed around. This was incredibly dangerous. Kale's mind raced—*What should I do? She's not consenting to this procedure. I have to tell the doctor to stop*—until he realized, *They can't stop. The abortion is almost completed, and if she keeps moving she's going to hurt herself.*

He cringed at the thought that if there had been an antichoicer in the room they would have had a field day. But the reality was, there was nothing else to do. Now this had to happen. She had had most of the abortion. The most important thing was to make sure that her uterus wasn't going to get punctured.

He had to try to help her be still. He cupped her shoulders in his hands and locked eyes with her, making contact with her in a way that would seem foreign outside of a medical scenario. "You have to do this." He captured her attention by getting in her space so that he was the only thing that she could see. "I'm so sorry this hurts, but you're going to finish … Because you have to. You're not the first person who has done this, and you won't be the last. Lots of people have done it before you and you can do it, too. You're really strong, you're doing a great job."

She nodded and cried into his hands, and in another thirty seconds it was all over. She thanked him for helping her get through it. She was glad she made it, even though it was so uncomfortable.

Kale leans his head on the window; the pressure of the

cold glass feels good. His activist background taught him a lot about political rhetoric and representation, what it means to care about people on a macro level. It taught him what justice looks like and what we all need to do to make it happen. It didn't tell him this. He didn't know about the stories.

Direct-care work means that you are entrenched in the narrative of another person: you're getting down low into the details of your client's life. How these stories get digested is hard to anticipate for many new doulas—an overarching theme in our interviews is that people feel compelled toward this work from some innate, unnameable place. We repeatedly hear accounts of doulas being told that they are "mothering," that they are "caregivers," and that they are drawn to this role because they want to be able to be the change they are trying to create. Direct practice means that you are not grasping only through theory—you have something tangible and powerful in front of you every day.

"The sharing of a story is a cultural strategy that has been used forever," says Aimee Thorne-Thomsen, a longtime leader in the reproductive justice movement and advisor to the Doula Project. "Sharing [stories] is how we pass down our values, teach our community how to navigate this world. So when you are in an abortion context, it actually starts to open things up. The more we talk, the more we have others sharing back."

As doulas, stories become a part of who we are, and it's not always a comfortable or easy balance. On one hand, we are bearing witness to someone else's experience. On the other, that experience gets interpolated by the caregiver—us—so that it become ours, too, though from a different angle. We think a lot about Sayantani DasGupta's article "Narrative Humility" when it comes to story sharing—where we define empathy as the acknowledgement of how much we don't know, rather than the arrogant projection of what we think we "get." The moment we feel comfortable saying that we know someone else's story is the moment we must realize we're actually being very egocentric: all we are seeing is ourselves.

We do not want to assume the texture of our client's story—how it was for her in the moment. But she was a part of our lives as much as we were a part of hers. Thorne-Thomsen points out that there is a symbiotic relationship of vulnerability in sharing a story. The power of story, she says, "is a breaking of isolation. There is an opportunity to build community with someone else and make yourself vulnerable at a time when other people may not be ready. It requires someone who is sharing to be brave, and then it's an invitation for you to be brave back."

It also requires you—as the listener, as the person who is bearing witness to the story—to be vulnerable and giving. You become, as Thorne-Thomsen calls it, a "story-holder." You are letting down your guard, to be soft and open with another person. Kale often thinks about the tension surrounding the words "vulnerable" and "resilient." He says, "It's usually that people, especially organizers, don't want others to be characterized as vulnerable; they want them to be resilient. I understand why, but when people need to go to the doctor, there are usually degrees of vulnerability. You are sick. You are hurt. You are vulnerable. One-on-one, everyone is complicated and messy. You do the work, and you see people who are crying and scared."

And resiliency, Kale reminds us, does not negate vulnerability. "People are both," he says.

Vicki encounters "the business of birth doula work" when she first starts out. She takes a fairly circuitous route to becoming a birth doula after quitting her job in food science following the birth of her son. She attends a birth doula class at random in an effort to "put herself out there" and "find something new" after years of being a stay-at-home mom. Like Kale, she has no idea of the impact it will have on her. She finds a training session, and she finds her heart.

Vicki lives in a more suburban part of New York, where many of the birth doula groups err on the side of "posh." She has been in touch with the Doula Project for a while but is not yet sure if she is interested in doing full-spectrum work, even though she is pro-choice. She shrugs. "I guess I just thought birth work was my calling."

So she begins her birth doula career with one of those aforementioned posh, business-modeled groups. She encounters loads of paying clients and a blinding professional gloss over everything. It is not her cup of tea. These are not the clients who she feels really need the help, nor does she like the business side of it.

The final straw comes at the intersection of this group and one of the major birth doula certifying organizations.

Vicki is working with a client with preeclampsia—a common but at times very urgent blood pressure issue that can arise during pregnancy. Rather than calling Vicki, the client announces on Facebook that she is going to have an emergency C-section (this, for the record, is not a nice thing to do to your doula).

Vicki immediately rushes to the hospital. She is there for hours after the cesarean birth, supporting her client through grieving being unable to have the birth she ideally wanted, and going with her to visit her baby in the neonatal intensive care unit (NICU). After, when Vicki calls the certifying organization, she is told that her client's birth "doesn't count." The woman on the phone quips gently: "That's so nice that you helped her. But that's not supporting a birth as a doula."

"Screw this," Vicki says.

She decides to take the plunge into full-spectrum doula work and is grateful that the Doula Project does not look to certification as the gold standard—honestly, many doula programs don't. Many of the doulas in the Doula Project never bother to become certified for their own personal reasons and because as an organization, we don't charge money for our service. It is a personal decision. We respect whether someone certifies or doesn't certify. We see that the need for doulas outweighs the often-prohibitive benefits of certification, so we don't mandate it. Vicki remembers that conversation well. "At that point, after meeting the Doula Project I saw that certification was for or could be for doulas who are choosing to be 'business doulas' and not 'activist doulas.' [I had] the feeling that what I want[ed] to do with my life [was] be an activist doula."

People decide to go into doula work for a wide variety of reasons, but most doula trainings also have curricula built around starting a business. It's certainly useful to know about so as to have the option, but that's not the route we went, nor is it the path that a lot of the doulas who are attracted to our project take. Vicki defines being an "activist doula" as being a doula that serves the community regardless of cost, especially emphasizing those individuals who wouldn't be able to access doulas easily otherwise. In the words of another activist doula, Chanel Porchia-Albert of Ancient Song Doula Services in Brooklyn: "We want to offer doulas to the people who have never even heard of what a doula is."

Vicki leads our birth doula program, which is no small undertaking. She mentors the majority of the new doulas in the Doula Project, which amounts to countless phone calls at all hours of the day and night, and many hours spent listening to doulas' questions and experiences in cafes. Beyond that, she oversees the three prongs of our program. One is the Doula Project partnership with a legal advocacy group called the Bronx Defenders, a program Vicki oversees with doula Symone, that assists parents who are at risk of losing their children to the foster-care system. Vicki also oversees our partnership with the midwives on City Hospital's labor and delivery floor, where doulas work in twelve-hour shifts. Finally, she coordinates the requests for birth doulas that come in through our web form.

She is proud of the "full-spectrum" aspect of our work:

I feel it makes our birth program unique, in New York if not in the country. There's a variety of programs in New

York where new doulas can volunteer to support people for a low stipend or for free. I think the tradition is to attend a couple volunteer births and then go into business. But one of the things that is very unique about this program is that our doulas do this because they are activists and want to do this kind of work. They're not just trying to gain experience; they're not going to go off and do something else. This is the way they want to be doulas.

Vicki's label of "activist doula" is meant to be somewhat tongue-in-cheek, but it feels apt, because so many of the doulas who identity as "full-spectrum" began first as activists. The marriage of the two means that your ability to speak on a macro level becomes tinged with the stories of your clients, these strangers who—as Whitney said in an earlier chapter—were completely alien to you, and you to them, maybe a week before. You are marked by your clients and by their stories, which have taken on a life of their own inside of you. You don't know where to put these stories. You do know that speaking theoretically, as is often expected when talking organizing or policy, makes you feel defensive, and you're not sure why.

Partially, it is burnout in interfacing with the bitter reality of the care you're fighting for. Part of it is that it's easier in some ways to find your path into direct care than it is to find your path out. And yet, it is primarily doulas—not providers or traditional activists—who are organizing around full-spectrum care.

Midwife Danika points to the politics around abortion as a primary culprit in keeping birthing care and abortion care somewhat separated, at least in providers' political conversation. "People don't want to touch abortion with a ten-foot pole. It's as if we can pretend if women don't get abortions that much, then we don't have to feel bad about not taking care of them. As a group of doctors and midwives . . . If you're uncomfortable with it, or you think it will ruffle feathers, or you don't want to do it yourself, then you just ignore it. I don't really understand morally or ethically how that's okay and how that continues to be propagated."

She says it goes right down to provider education. While everyone is taught how to deliver a baby, most OBs and midwives are not taught how to perform abortions. "If that's not even there as a given, it's never going to be pulled through your practice. We start at a baseline of ignoring the possibility that abortion can be a part of a woman's healthcare. Full-spectrum [care] gets lost because of this political environment surrounding something that is completely normal."

She adds that midwives aren't able to lead this movement while they're still fighting for their own legitimacy in a lot of hospitals and practices. "I'm fighting for my patient's autonomy just to get up and walk around during her labor. These small issues are huge. If we are not respecting a woman's bodily autonomy . . . where do we even start?"

We also can't shake off the chronic potential for trauma and mistakes that haunt medical providers. Providers, especially doctors during residency, are often just trying to keep their heads above water so that they have a chance to potentially enjoy their lives. Being an abortion provider is hard enough as it is without the added risk of "outing" oneself and living with the fear of being attacked.

Doulas are able to bridge both sides of the activist-service binary, and they work within story-based care to project outward toward a larger movement. It means that those of us who take on this work have stumbled upon another ethical obligation—to find ways to talk about this work with respect to our clients, yet to be aware of boundaries and to unflinchingly bear witness when needed. We need to always be malleable: able to conform to what the medical system needs, while being aware of how we can shift, change, challenge, and support it and then communicate it back to the broader movement. Thorne-Thomsen underscores this:

> [You] aren't doulas on a national level, you are doulas in a community, in a hospital, in a neighborhood clinic. [You are] local service providers—and that connection of local to national is critical. The people that doulas are serving are not the same people that policy makers are thinking of when they are passing some of these awful laws. It's the culture shift . . . doulas aren't just talking about the good abortion story or the uncomplicated one but multiple stories that run the gamut. In sharing those stories it complicates things in ways that are important. Hopefully, it also allows us to open up the doors around abortion but also around pregnancy. To me, doulas complicate the conversation in the best way possible.

In committing to a direct-care practice, we've pledged to working within the fine fibers of the stories of our clients. People feel an intrinsic desire to be seen and for their stories to be validated. Our job is to do that but also to help wipe tears, give hugs, and celebrate sometimes. We look at pictures of our clients' children, we stroke hair, and we receive love from one another at times when it feels like no one else would be able to understand what our day has been like. And how can we explain it? How can we be sure of who wants to hear it?

Kale reflects on this on his train ride back home, the dawning understanding that direct care cannot always be put into words. Vicki charges through her doula organizing, a story always in the back of her mind.

How to Build
a Full-Spectrum Model

A mini chapter—featuring other doula organizations from around the country—filled with important lessons we learned from an organizational standpoint while starting the Doula Project. This chapter is especially geared toward anyone who wishes to become a full-spectrum doula or start their own group.

Be Patient

This is one of the "best practices" we have to share: be patient. Full-spectrum work is intricate, and it takes time to develop. The first year of the Doula Project was spent creating a mission statement and putting together the bones of a practice model. It's important to note that before we were fully engaged in the clinical work, constructing a comprehensive organizational model was difficult. In addition, it took us months to find a clinic to partner with. While other doula groups have established sites more quickly, every group and community moves at a different pace.

We recommend researching clinics and hospitals in your area as well as looking into the pregnancy needs in your community. This is also a great time to start talking to other doula groups around the country to see what their best practices are. Try not to get frustrated . . . most organizations take a solid year to get off the ground!

Promote Your Work

Promoting your work and garnering enthusiasm for full-spectrum doula care in your community is something you can do before you get into a clinic or start working with clients. No matter what kind of doula practice you want your organization to have, networking and promoting your idea is a great way to get the world excited about your mission and your message.

We recommend going to social and reproductive justice meetings in your community, speaking on panels at conferences, or organizing your own local talks and gatherings. We spoke publicly about our work for a year before we found a clinic and, ultimately, met our first clinic partner while speaking at a movement meeting organized by Exhale and the Guttmacher Institute.

The Bay Area Doula Project has also had success promoting the full-spectrum model through their self-organized Salon Series. According to Poonam Dreyfus-Pai, the series was "a monthly conversation about something related to full-spectrum work or reproductive justice in general. So we would have activists or artists come in and talk about their work and have larger dialogues about connections between political events that were happening and the work we do. It was a great way to bring people into the work that full-spectrum doulas were doing. And also broaden our reach a little, like a clinic would hear about us and want to work with us."

Talk to Other Full-Spectrum Doula Groups

More than a dozen similar doula organizations exist around the United States, and they all have invaluable information and lessons to share about what works and what doesn't. There is no reason to do this work in isolation!

Nafeesa Dawoodbhoy of the SPIRAL Collective in Minneapolis, Minnesota, says, "Get in touch with other full-spectrum groups! Research full-spectrum groups around the country, find a model you like, and seek direct advice. Don't reinvent the wheel. We are all here to offer our resources and share them with each other."

Sarah Whedon of the Boston Doula Project says, "As much as possible connect with, follow on social media, and talk directly with folks who are already leading or who've had the experience of starting up full-spectrum doula groups. A lot of groups have wisdom to share as well as written materials and other resources. It's very helpful to know how others have addressed problems and opportunities—plus other full-spectrum doulas are just really cool people to know."

Dreyfus-Pai created a network that keeps many of these doula groups connected. She says:

I put out a call on social media and asked all my doula

friends, "If you're in a doula group and interested in being part of some coordinated body, let me know." I wanted to talk to people directly about what they thought the need was and what they wanted to see happen. And what they wanted was some sort of regular meeting with other doula groups. . . . They wanted to know about how groups trained volunteers and fostered relationships with clinics and other partners. They also wanted to just reach out and support other groups as they came up, kind of paying it forward. So I worked with, at the time, nine groups from eight states, and we created a national network of full-spectrum doula groups.

Be Professional When Approaching Potential Partners

First impressions mean *a lot* when speaking to potential clinic partners. Be open, flexible, cheerful, and informed about how to integrate the doula role. Doulas are often the sunshine in any medical room, and you want to show them that from the start. You also want to show them that you have ideas about how to engage doulas in their clinic while being respectful of the standards of practice they already have in place.

Don't Rush to Get Incorporated

Before getting incorporated, make sure you can do the actual doula work first, that you have leadership and volunteers in place, and a steady client base. Getting a 501(c)(3)—non-profit tax status—is time-consuming, and your efforts will be better spent on programming in the early days of your organization. You are valuable and legitimate even if you are not recognized as an official nonprofit entity by the government.

We waited four years to get incorporated. We had already served thousands of clients and partnered with three clinic sites. Even though we are now able to have a bigger budget and fundraise more widely, we still operate in a similar grassroots fashion to what we did in our early days.

Some groups never plan to get incorporated and have devised other structures. Janna Blair Slack, a full-spectrum doula in Oregon and the founder of the LA Doula Project, says:

> Depending on what's going on in your area, consider whether it's worth doing all the work to start your *own* organization, or if it would be a better use of everyone's time to partner with an existing clinic or organization and go directly into doing the work—rather than going through the time-suck that is setting up a 501(c)(3) or other organizational structures. If you partner with an existing (c)(3), you can often become a "project" of that organization, granting you a tax ID number for fundraising, and sometimes even administrative and accounting support. Build on the structures in your community that already exist, if at all possible.

Be in the Clinic Every Day

Seriously. Make the clinic staff think they can't do the work without you. If you are the person launching the program, we recommend being present in the clinic for at least a month before you train anyone else. This way you understand the role intensely. No matter how broad your knowledge base on abortion, birth, or adoption, every facility operates differently. If you do not have a flexible schedule—and most of us don't—think about bringing on a small crew of doulas to help you launch.

Be Open to Different Practice Models

There are several different ways to engage in abortion doula care. Some doula groups have had success in supporting people through medical abortions in their homes. Others leave cards at clinics for clients who want to be accompanied on the day of their procedure. If your heart is set on partnering with a clinic, these are good ways to gain credibility in your community and build relationships in order to get there.

In 2011 Dreyfus-Pai left the Doula Project and joined the Bay Area Doula Project in California. She was committed to the clinic model she was practicing in New York City, but when she got out west, she and fellow organizational leaders realized they needed to try something different:

> The hope was to use the Doula Project model to set up in clinics, and we thought since the Bay Area has such a culture of doula presence—particularly birth—that having abortion doulas would be not only obvious but very accepted, the Bay area being fairly progressive. We were met with the response, 'Oh, abortion doulas sound won-

derful, but we don't want to be the clinic that is your pilot or guinea pig, so try it out somewhere else, let us know how it goes, and we will be in touch.' It wasn't that they were opposed to the idea, they just didn't want to put their clinic[s] on the line. . . . We started doing trainings for how to do [medical] abortion support at home and really built that out. We talked to a lot of home-birth doulas on how to create that process and what it looks like in someone's home. So we created an eight-hour shift training. [Clients] would call the Bay Area Project, and we'd connect them to a doula, and they would have a phone conversation to get a sense of what the [client] wanted out of the experience. And then they go to their home, and have a buddy, another doula, available by phone.

Create Local Partnerships Beyond Clinics

Reach out to organizations that work directly with mothers and pregnant people. Not only will this create access for more people to have doulas, it will also create a supportive network of allies.

Dreyfus-Pai explains how the Bay Area Doula Project created a crucial partnership with ACCESS Women's Health Justice, a local reproductive health hotline and abortion fund that provides multiple support services to people who need abortions. "We officially approached them about partnering and adding doulas to the list of services they offer through their practical support network. So now when people want an abortion doula, they call ACCESS, and they say they want an abortion doula. All ACCESS volunteers are trained [by the Bay Area Doula Project] to do doula work, if they want to."

Remember, You Are a Guest

We've said it before, but here it is again: whether you are a doula in a clinic, hospital, birthing center, or someone's home, you are a guest. Follow the rules of whatever space you are in, if you want to be allowed back. If you disagree with something you see, be strategic about how you communicate this (i.e., not during a procedure) and whom you communicate it to. Pick your battles. Not everything is worth fighting for. It may go against your personal beliefs, but keep in mind that medical settings are very different from activist settings, for better or worse. And you want to be invited back in. The clients need you there. We have partnered with clinics in the past that were not a good fit for us. We came up with a strategy for pulling out and were transparent about our reasons. While we finished out our time at these clinics, however, we abided by all of their policies.

Be Strategic about Recruitment

When recruiting, don't assume the activist or the person educated in "social justice speak" will be the best doula. While that is an excellent foundation to come in with, don't overlook people who aren't as familiar with it. In addition to people who know the language of abortion rights or birth justice, we recommend looking for people who have direct-care experience or personal stories that connect them to the work. Spread the word widely over LISTSERVs and social media and to friends and colleagues. Table at health fairs or community college events. Hang flyers in bodegas and grocery stores.

Grayson Morris, an abortion doula at Open Umbrella in Asheville, North Carolina, says, "You will be surprised at how many people want to help. Keep searching for them. You will find them!"

Always Do an Application and Interview Process

Let's be real. Clinics are under attack. If you are working in a clinic, they trust you to bring in trustworthy people. If you are working with birth or abortion clients independently, your clients trust you to provide them with trusting care-givers. Before accepting them into your organization, we recommend you should meet with potential doulas and conduct a rigorous interview. Due to the sensitive and confidential nature of our role, clinics appreciate the extra screening. Always remember, your organization's name is on this work. It only takes one person to mess it up for you. Nearly ten years in, with partnerships almost as old, we still take this concern seriously. If you give yourself the time to find the right people, it will ultimately bring you peace of mind.

Have a Personnel Policy

No matter how grassroots you are, having a personnel policy is important. Everyone needs to be on the same page and held accountable in the same way. Clinics and clients rely on you to be present at every shift. The policy will support your organization as it expands and as you take on more volunteers. People come into doula care with the best of intentions, but the truth is, this work is mostly unpaid, and for some volunteers, it is just one stop on the way to other career paths. We recommend having volunteers sign a memorandum of understanding stating that they will take a certain number of shifts (the Doula Project asks for two) each month for at least a year. Dreyfus-Pai says:

> Volunteer management is hard work. If you're managing a group of volunteers, know that your job is basically [to be] a wrangler. You are asking people to give up their time and energy—presumably for something they're interested in—and people still won't part with them easily. Managing volunteers requires clear guidelines, some firmness, a lot of love and appreciation, and people you can gripe to when it gets frustrating. It can feel thankless, but you're helping people do work that matters to them. And if people are not fulfilling their requirements—it's okay to cut them loose. You can do that gently and with understanding, but it's important to have standards—clients are expecting a certain quality of care, and other volunteers who show up 100 percent should be able to see that their peers [and] teammates are pulling equal weight.

Training Matters

It's hard to predict how a doula will respond to a situation with a client, whether in a clinic or in someone's home. We recommend you spend time training every doula both in the classroom and on-site with a client to help the doula avoid missteps. Recognize that doulas will require different levels and quantities of training—everyone arrives with unique experiences and varied sets of skills. Medical staff and clients will give feedback about the doulas, so developing the highest quality of training possible is more than worth the time and energy.

Just as important, training builds confidence in the doulas. Many doulas are new to the way full-spectrum organizations operate, and a strong foundation of education on their role is extremely important to them. A thought-provoking training is also an important way for doulas to reflect on their feelings about abortion before going into the procedure room.

Abortion doula Mallory Mahoney remembers her Doula Project training well:

> Training teaches us how to understand other people and ourselves . . . I think it's one of the most valuable things I've gotten from the Doula Project, that initial abortion training. I still talk about it with people in my life. It taught me to reevaluate my views and question, "Am I really okay supporting people having abortions?" I always thought I was, but I think it's important to really reflect on it, rather than it just being drilled into us. It's more than an ideology. There is power in remembering or realizing why you feel a certain way. And there were questions [at the training] that were not easy to answer.

Experiment with Different Models of Leadership

There are several different decision-making and leadership

models being used by doula groups all over the country, from consensus-based leadership groups to directorships to codirectorships. Study the different models, think about what kind of organization you want to run, and reflect on your own personality and what you feel capable of. Be open to changing your leadership model if it is not working—and, remember, there are benefits and drawbacks to every model.

Reach out to other groups to learn more about different models so you can decide what might align best with your mission. Whatever you try, be kind to yourself and give other potential leaders the benefit of the doubt. It's not easy work, and many of you may just be learning how to be leaders. Be open to bringing in outside facilitators to help you move through difficult leadership transitions.

In the first two years of the Doula Project, we operated as codirectors. As the work expanded, we reflected on the kind of organization we wanted to be ideologically, and we changed to a leadership circle with a team of doulas making consensus-based decisions and running daily operations.

Plan for Burnout and Attrition

Most of this work is unpaid or underpaid, time-consuming, and emotionally challenging. Anticipate fatigue. Burnout is common in direct care, period. When bringing on new doulas, recruit more than you think you need. In addition to the burnout factor, some attrition will naturally happen after training, especially when your partner sites have lengthy volunteer processes or people realize they don't actually have the time to commit.

Many doulas we interviewed for this book mentioned that burnout came less from client work and more from supporting other doulas or running organizations. If you are a leader and ready to resign your position, create a long-term exit strategy and transition plan to give future leaders a chance to learn your role.

Slack says:

> It can be physically and mentally exhausting to hold the container for all the enthusiasm and passion that come[s] pouring out of people in the founding of a new doula collective or group. If the person holding the container burns out and others haven't had an active role, the entire project can fall apart. Set up accountability frameworks and timelines but also respect the nonlinear doula way of doing things. Trust that things will get done even if there isn't an Excel spreadsheet.

Dreyfus-Pai also advises, "Make an exit plan—it's not necessary for you to be the wrangler for the rest of your life! It will help you put your best work and self forward, knowing that you don't have to be in one specific role forever. The work will continue, for you and the group, and though that may take different paths or shapes, that's all ok."

Let Your Clients Lead You

A common refrain in social work and justice practice is, "Meet your clients where they are." You will likely enter doula care with a certain number of assumptions about what your clients need or how they might identify with their situation. That's normal if you are new to doula care. The important thing is to adapt to your clients' needs within the bounds of your mission. Listen to and learn from your clients. They will lead your organization where it needs to go in terms of direct-care programming.

When we formed, we called ourselves the Abortion Doula Project, assuming that all of our clients would identify with "having an abortion." We soon learned that we were supporting people experiencing fetal losses and those who—for religious, cultural, or personal safety reasons—did not or could not use the word "abortion." We quickly learned to use reflective language and, ultimately, changed our name to the Doula Project after a few months in the clinic.

Early in our birth doula practice, we also had a client who did not identify as a woman. This prompted us to begin referring to all of our clients as "pregnant people," something we had been considering for political reasons anyway. In addition, while establishing our programming, we made detailed plans to provide postabortion care, such as helping a client get home or following up by phone. We assumed this would become a big piece of our mission. It turned out that our clients didn't lead us there.

But Know That You Can't Be Everything to Everyone

Doulas often need to relearn this several times over. Why? Because we want to help *everyone*.

Before you begin, it's important to do a community needs assessment and also ponder what kind of work really interests you. Once your program takes off, medical departments and organizations that reach beyond the scope of pregnancy-care practice may approach you.

At one point the Doula Project considered attending colposcopies and IUD insertions at the request of one of our clinics. Due to our capacity and our desire to remain directly focused on pregnancy care, we decided to stick to our mission of pregnancy only. In the first year of our organization we also thought about creating an affiliate model of doula groups around the country. In the end we felt it would be better for us and for other groups to simply provide guides for starting up, and trainings where we could.

We considered a branch of the Doula Project that would escort transgender clients to medical appointments. Again, we realized we didn't have the capacity and that another group of individuals may be better suited to that role. To that end, we recently supported the launch and training of the Trans Buddy program in Nashville, Tennessee, the first group ever to utilize a similar doula-based model of care to support transgender people through medical appointments.

Finally, don't overcommit yourself to the spectrum of care. If you want to practice the full spectrum—birth, abortion, adoption, fetal loss—make sure you have the capacity. Some groups have opted to take on a piece of the spectrum—abortion only or birth only—and are clear about their roles and who they are. Others—like the Doula Project—have started with only one aspect (in our case, abortion) and then expanded to the full spectrum as they gained more capacity.

Dreyfus-Pai says:

> Understand that what works in one place may not work in another—the political landscape, the number of providers, the restrictions on a clinic or hospital, the existing presence of doulas (full-spectrum or otherwise), and the number of committed team members all shape the process of creating a doula group, and these will all differ by location. So, learn from other groups, and also know that you don't have to do it exactly the way that others have.

Allow the Organization to Change, but Follow a Road Map

Just because something worked in the past doesn't mean that's what is best for it now. Community needs and partnerships may change. Leadership may turn over and new ideas may come in. Be open to adjusting the style and scope of your work. Still, don't get caught up in rapid change with each new iteration of leadership. That can lead to organizational instability and confusion from the rest of the field about your message and contribution. Operating under a three- to five-year strategic plan is a great way to ensure long-term goals are met while also reevaluating the work on a regular basis. We recommend bringing in outside facilitators to help with the strategic-planning process.

Finally, doula care is an interesting mix of the static and the dynamic. The job is simple, even unchanging: continuous emotional, physical, and educational support. Yet the ways in which doula care is transforming pregnancy care are incredibly dynamic. Many full-spectrum doulas are at the cusp of this change. Anyone starting their own doula group is entering into a powerful and revolutionary moment.

Conclusion
Always a Doula

When we set out to write this book, our intention was to let people into the world of full-spectrum doulas. We wanted to show what it means to exist in this role on a daily basis. We wanted to paint an accurate and nuanced portrait of how people come to their decisions around pregnancy outcomes and how doulas support those decisions.

In conducting oral histories with doulas, we tried to go in with very little agenda:

"Take us back to the time before you became a doula: What was your life like, what were you doing?"

"Tell us about your role as if we'd never heard the word *doula* before."

"Close your eyes and think about the work: What do you see, smell, hear, touch?"

We believed that the history and politics of abortion and birth care as we saw them would naturally emerge through our research and interviews, and that the experiences of the millions of people who get pregnant each year would be well represented in these stories. What we found instead was a collection of stories about the toll of caregiving, the deep love involved in supporting others through important transitions, the healing effects of this work, the guilt we carry for having feelings at all, the fear we hold in taking from our clients' stories when we tell our own, and the fractures in each of our hearts.

After several oral histories we began to panic: there were too many stories of trauma. Was this going to be an inaccurate portrayal of our work, our doulas, and our clients? We put our heads together and brainstormed doulas we knew who had attended "happy births." We began to reflect on our own personal stories—we had certainly been to very few happy births. What was a happy birth anyway? Even the happy births aren't necessarily happy for the doula.

We turned to similar professional fields for guidance and read creative nonfiction works by other direct-care workers. They told intense stories of caregiving, stories that didn't always have happy endings, stories in which they didn't always "like" their clients, stories where their feelings were shameful, and where their guts were left wrenched. Through this we realized that the best story we could tell was the one closest to our hearts. Hearts that had been broken and then put back together by this work. Hearts that came to the work already wounded and found a safe space to heal. Whenever we felt stuck or afraid to take this book to a place it needed to go—whether because of the political landscape or because we didn't want to expose a part of ourselves—we went back to our roots as doulas. These roots have told us to be nonjudgmental, unconditionally supportive, and, above all, honest. The world doesn't need more sugarcoating: it needs to see what we see.

Of the many doulas we spoke to throughout the process of writing this book, some are still practicing in the context of pregnancy, and some are not. The philosophy of doula care, however, stays with them in everything they do: listening to and supporting others, holding space, being kind. For most, being a doula is not only a practice, but also an identity they carry with them wherever they go.

Kat Broadway, who continues to volunteer at Planned Parenthood every month, says:

> I work at a cardiac unit [as a nurse], but I still am a doula at work. . . . One day I was walking down the hall, and a patient who was not my patient [was] screaming, and I went into the room. They were dressing this horrible wound from a pacemaker extraction. A four-by-four-by-four wound. She was screaming in pain, and I just was a doula. I dropped everything I was doing, went in, and got down on my knees. I took her hand and let her scream. I rubbed her head.

Mallory Mahoney, a practicing abortion doula and social work graduate student, says:

> The Doula Project gave me the opportunity to build on something I had inside me that I wasn't able to get to before. It's an identity. This is who I am. I'm doing something for others—I'm not just living for myself. There's

a level of elevation and self-actualization that can happen because this is a relationship I'm experiencing without it being about me, and there is something enlightening about that. It makes the world feel larger. You're out there experiencing other people's worlds, even if briefly. It's a privilege to do that and know someone in that way. We all just want to know each other in a real way, I think. And you are getting to know someone in a real way in that moment. If I hadn't become a doula . . . I would have a lot more to learn about life.

Poonam Dreyfus-Pai is not currently practicing as a doula but holds this identity close to whatever she does. Growing up, she saw her mom serve in a doula-like role in her mostly Indian community, providing emotional support to women going through challenging transitions. "This is my connection; it isn't just with these [doula] groups but as part of me through my heritage. That is what enables me to identify as a full-spectrum doula. I don't want the name to mean anything and everything, but the essence of doula work can exist in a lot of different places."

Cofounder and full-spectrum doula Miriam Zoila Pérez, who returned to the Doula Project several years after its inception to serve as an abortion doula, confirms this sentiment, "It has shaped how I see what it means to support another human being. Whether it's my friends, or my family members, or other people I encounter, the principle that often the best thing I can do is simply witness another's experience, validate their feelings, and lend a supportive hand has been an incredible guide to me in all my interactions."

This has been the story of the Doula Project. It's the story our doulas wanted to tell—the one we wanted you to know. These are the stories that moved us and changed us as doulas and as people. We raised several questions at the beginning of the book, wondering: What are we? Where do we belong? What do we want to become?

The process of writing this book helped us expose the very nature of our role, that we don't fit into any neat packages and that we don't need to. We are an organization on the fringe. We are doulas.

Afterword

A word about the significance of this book is in order. Often when new terms enter the public domain, or old terms take on new meanings, the challenge is first definitional—followed by the challenge of justification. Such was the task for the coauthors of this book. Since the rescue of the term "doula" from antiquity (where it was primarily used to describe a nonmedically trained birth attendant present in support of a laboring woman), women now have possibilities during labor that all but disappeared with the medicalization of childbirth. Amidst our current social preoccupation with optimizing outcome for the labor process—defined by some as minimizing litigious concerns—the default to crude measures of infant mortality and or maternal morbidity has distracted us from the central players in pregnancy: *women*.

This book seeks to rescue us from that myopia. Lauren and Mary rigorously establish doulas and their training as an innovative approach to achieving the same goal of optimal outcomes, while also restoring women to their central place in the birthing process—as ethics and common sense demand. The result is a birth experience that is more humane and firmly rooted in the reality of an individual pregnant person, even when medicalization intervenes.

What is unique about this book? So much. It brings precision to the term "doula." It makes the case for the role that doulas can play in empowering women to achieve the reproductive outcomes that they desire beyond birth—for example, nurturing management of a miscarriage or a supported abortion to meet a woman's desire to avoid involuntary parenthood. Magnificently, this book frames doula practice as a calling for the practitioner and puts forth the notion of such support as an *entitlement*—not a luxury—for women. The authors skillfully deploy this frame to guide any logistical concerns for would-be doulas about how to become one, while insisting that doula services be democratized to the point of being available to all women who need or choose them—irrespective of ability to pay. The doulas refuse to allow their practice to become a boutique service consumable only by those who can afford it. Rather, they position doula practice to be value-added support to women, even when we cannot alter the other determinants of health in her life.

In *The Doulas* the authors serve as the "doulas to the doula" by enabling those who see the value of this practice to explore the best way of availing themselves to the doula mission. The authors cover the art of doula-ing in a comprehensive way—which makes sense given that the core value of a doula practice is based on a holistic approach to reproduction and its continuum as a function of healthy sexuality and decision-making. Incisive sections such as "How to Talk to the Press," "How to Self-Care," and "Activist Practice" provide instructions on how to build the capacity for long-term, thriving doula practice and speak to the brilliant, thoughtful, and comprehensive approach of these authors. Anyone responsible for training aspiring practitioners for their craft would do well to model their work after this seminal text.

—WILLIE PARKER, MD, MPH
Birmingham, Alabama
March 2016

Glossary

ABORTION DOULA A doula who attends abortions. The Doula Project was the first organization to formalize this role—though nurses, counselors, and volunteers have acted in a similar capacity for years. We have partnered with abortion clinics to be with clients during procedures so that our doulas are fully integrated into clinic care. Doulas meet clients in the waiting room before procedures, provide support during the abortion itself, and assist in the recovery room after. All of the doulas in the Doula Project are trained to support clients through first and second trimester surgical abortions and to manage miscarriages. Abortion doulas also attend medical abortions, typically outside of the clinic setting.

ADOPTION PLAN When speaking about the process of adoption, we use language that centers the birth parent with whom we work. Rather than saying the client "gave the baby up for adoption" we say the client "made an adoption plan."

This language helps the client feel more in control of her decision and also reflects the values of "open adoption," which allows the birth parent to continue having a relationship with the child—if so desired—after the adoption takes place.

BIRTH CONTRACT A document that outlines the roles and responsibilities of both the doula and the client. An example from a Doula Project contract: a doula will agree to attend at least one prenatal meeting and a client will agree to inform the doula as soon as she goes into labor.

BIRTH DOULA A doula who is present for a client's labor and delivery. Birth doulas will often meet clients prior to their due date. Doula Project doulas are asked to meet with their clients once or twice before the birth, if possible, to review the birth plan, and offer childbirth education if necessary. The client will usually call the doula when her labor begins, and the two will decide when and where it's best for the doula to meet the client. Whether the doula meets the client at home or at the hospital, she will stay until the baby is born. Following the birth, it is common practice for doulas to help clients initiate breastfeeding. They will also meet with their clients at least once after the birth for a postpartum visit.

BIRTH DOULA TRAINING ORGANIZATIONS These groups provide new doulas with a set of core skills to draw on as they begin their practice. The most well-known organizations on the national level are Doulas of North America (DONA), Childbirth and Postpartum Professional Association (CAPPA), toLabor, Childbirth International, and the International Center for Traditional Childbearing Full Circle Doula Training (ICTC). There are also community-based doula training organizations, such as Ancient Song Doula Services in New York City. Many doulas are also trained by apprenticing with midwives as birth assistants.

BIRTH PARENT *or* **BIRTH MOTHER** When speaking of the person who gives birth to the child, we refer to that person as the "birth parent" or "birth mother."

CESAREAN SECTION (C-SECTION) The delivery of a baby through a surgical cut in the abdominal and uterine walls. C-sections can be planned prior to labor or initiated during labor. Because it is a major abdominal surgery, recovery time can take over two weeks. While C-sections can have lifesaving results for mom and baby, they have become used more frequently than medically advised. In the last decade, the rate reached over 30 percent of all births in the country—contrasted with the World Health Organization's recommendation that only 10 to 15 percent of births be delivered by cesarean.

CASTOR OIL Castor oil is better known as a laxative than a method of labor induction but has been used for years to help women naturally induce after their fortieth week. Some doulas believe that castor oil does bring on contractions, but it can also cause diarrhea and dehydration.

CHUCK An ultra-absorbent fabric pad used during medical procedures. A chuck is typically placed on the procedure table underneath the patient or on the surrounding floor to catch bodily fluids.

CONSCIOUS SEDATION A type of sedation employed to help clients relax and to reduce discomfort and anxiety during a first trimester abortion procedure. A combination of the medications Versed (to induce sedation) and fentanyl (to induce pain relief) is injected through an IV. Many clients remain awake with this type of sedation but may become drowsy and have little memory of the procedure. The effects of the sedation wear off quickly once the procedure is over. This method is the one most commonly used at our clinic sites, followed by local sedation.

COURT-ORDERED C-SECTION Sometimes (often for well-informed reasons) mothers disagree with doctors' advice and refuse to consent to cesarean surgery or other recommended medical interventions. On occasion, doctors have gone to the courts seeking to obtain an order permitting them to perform the surgery without the patient's consent or threatened such action as a way of coercing consent from the patient. Some courts have granted such orders and surgery has been performed over the patient's objections (and without consent). The weight of legal authority, however, holds that such orders violate constitutional rights. In addition, major medical organizations have clearly stated that threatening and seeking such orders violates patient rights and medical ethics.

DILATION AND CURETTAGE Commonly known as "D and C," this is a method of first trimester abortion in which the cervix is widened and the pregnancy is removed from the uterus through scraping or scooping with a metal instrument called a "sharp curette." D and C is rarely practiced today and has been largely replaced by manual vacuum aspiration (MVA) or electric suction aspiration (EVA) in the United States. In the medical community and the clinics we practice in, however, the term "D and C" typically refers to any first trimester surgical process where the cervix is dilated and the pregnancy is removed.

DILATION AND EVACUATION Commonly known as "D and E," this is a method of second trimester surgical abortion in which the cervix is widened and the pregnancy is evacuated from the uterus, using both forceps and suction. Because the pregnancy is larger than in the first trimester, laminaria sticks—tubes of sterile seaweed which absorb and expand to widen the cervix further—must be inserted. This widening process is done at our clinics at least one day prior to the abortion. Patients are typically placed under general anesthesia during a D and E but not during laminaria insertion. Doulas attend both laminaria insertions and the abortion itself.

DOULA The word doula is derived from ancient Greek and means "female slave." In the mid-twentieth century, it was popularly retranslated as "woman who serves." Doulas traditionally provide continuous emotional, physical, and informational support to women during labor and delivery. Today the term spans to support people across pregnancy outcomes as well as people who are dying or experiencing other major life transitions.

ELECTRIC VACUUM ASPIRATION (EVA) Similar to manual vacuum aspiration, EVA is a surgical procedure that uses a suction device to remove the pregnancy from the uterus. EVA uses an electric pump instead of a manual one and makes a louder sound than the MVA. Both instruments are similar in suction strength, and selection is usually based on provider preference and patient comfort. (The clinics our doulas practice in predominantly use either MVA or EVA for first trimester surgical abortions.)

EPIDURAL A regional anesthesia used during labor and C-sections, in which medication is injected through a catheter into the lower spine. The effect is that the body becomes numb from the waist down and some of the pain of contractions is relieved. While incredibly popular, epidurals have been known to adversely affect the baby's heart rate and can sometimes slow labor down.

FETAL HEART MONITOR A device used to measure the frequency and duration of contractions, as well as the heart rate of the fetus during labor. It is typically placed on the pregnant person's abdomen externally, over the area of the fetal heart.

FREESTANDING ABORTION CLINIC A medical facility that provides abortion services outside of a hospital setting. These can be public or private establishments. Planned Parenthood is an example of a freestanding clinic.

FULL-SPECTRUM DOULA A doula who provides continuous, compassionate support to clients during birth, abortion, adoption, miscarriage, stillbirth, or perinatal loss. The Doula Project developed this term as a way to describe the broad aspects of the work we do: support across the spectrum of pregnancy options and experiences.

HOLDING SPACE or HOLDING ENVIRONMENT A term originally coined by the pediatrician and psychoanalyst D. W. Winnicott, this refers to a metaphorical "space" that brings about a feeling of nurturance, calm, and safety for a client. This space can be created through soothing words, physical touch, and other body language, as well as through the fulfillment of a necessary role or transference for a client (i.e., a doula serving to hold some of her client's emotional pain).

LABOR INDUCTION Pregnant clients planning to terminate may elect to have an induction due to personal or religious preference, a medical concern, bureaucratic delay, or a desire to abort close to the legal limit. The first step of a labor induction is a lethal fetal injection (of either KCl or digoxin), initiated both for patient preference and to comply with the 2003 ban on one later-term abortion technique. From there, the client is instructed to go to the labor and delivery floor. Inductions are initiated through the use of medications to provoke labor, much like the medications used in a first trimester medical abortion but with higher doses. The client experiences labor contractions, often for many hours, and then gives birth and delivers the fetus and placenta. (Our doulas commonly attend inductions at City Hospital.)

LAMINARIA Thin rods or sticks made of seaweed that are placed inside the cervix to help safely expand it before an abortion. Anywhere from one to more than a dozen may be inserted, depending on the number of gestational weeks.

LOCAL SEDATION A type of sedation used during first trimester abortions in which the client is awake and able to feel some of what is happening during the procedure. Lidocaine is the most common type of anesthetic used. It is injected into the cervix and works as a numbing agent so that the cervix is more relaxed, and pain-producing nerve impulses are blocked. Lidocaine, however, does not help reduce the discomfort of cramping in the uterus.

MANUAL VACUUM ASPIRATION (MVA) The most common method of first trimester abortion. This procedure involves removing the pregnancy from the uterus with a handheld plastic aspirator that creates suction. Manual Vacuum Aspiration utilizes a less expensive instrument, is associated with less blood loss, and typically requires less pain medication than a traditional D and C.

MEDICAL ABORTION Also known as the "abortion pill," this is a method of pregnancy termination through the ingestion of misoprostol and mifepristone. It induces a process similar to a miscarriage. It is nonsurgical and is often taken within a client's own home, though clinic visits are required both before and after the pregnancy is passed. Medical abortion tends to be most effective in early pregnancy. (Our clinics offer the abortion pill to clients, though the Doula Project typically does not attend these abortions.)

MIDWIFE A trained medical professional who provides care to people during pregnancy and childbirth as well as primary reproductive healthcare. A midwife practices a client-centered and empowering model of maternity care that utilizes fewer medical interventions.

MUCOUS PLUG Commonly referred to as "bloody show," this is a gelatinous plug that seals the cervical canal and protects bacteria from entering the uterus during pregnancy. The mucous plug typically comes out in early labor as the cervix dilates.

NEW YORK STATE ABORTION POLICY Abortion is legal up to twenty-four weeks in New York State, and many procedures are at least partially covered by Medicaid. A licensed doctor is required to perform abortions in New York, and the state must abide by the policies set forth in several federal laws.

OB-GYN A trained physician (obstetrician and gynecologist) who specializes in reproductive healthcare, pregnancy, and childbirth, and performs the majority of surgical abortions in the United States.

OPEN ADOPTION The law that means—in a nutshell—that the birth parent has the right to keep in contact with the child, and the adoptive parent must agree to these terms. The birth parent also has the option to select the adoptive parents and meet them before the birth.

PALLIATIVE CARE or DEATH DOULA A doula who provides support to clients as they are about to pass on. The Doula Project does not explicitly identify as a death doula organization, but we have served in a similar role for our clients who have experienced miscarriages or stillbirth losses.

PITOCIN A common labor induction medication, Pitocin is a synthetic version of a hormone called "oxytocin" and functions by causing powerful uterine contractions to start, speed up, or induce labor. It doesn't necessarily help soften or open the cervix as quickly—the effect can be likened to squeezing a tube of toothpaste without taking the cap off. It is known to cause intense, painful contractions and often leads to greater use of pain medications, like the epidural.

PLACENTA ACCRETA This occurs during pregnancy when blood vessels and other parts of the placenta grow too deeply into the uterine wall, causing the placenta to remain in the womb after the birth of the baby and inducing severe maternal blood loss.

POSTPARTUM DOULA A doula who works with clients after the birth of their baby and in the weeks that immediately follow. Postpartum doulas have extensive knowledge of breastfeeding and newborn care and can help alleviate common anxieties for new parents. In addition, one of their primary functions is to help the client process the experience of her birth and tell her birth story. The Doula Project does not currently offer postpartum support beyond a single visit to the home in the week following the birth, but we consider it a crucial service for new parents. One organization doing incredible postpartum work is the Eugene, Oregon–based Daisy C.H.A.I.N.

PREGNANT PEOPLE A term we helped popularize to be inclusive of all people who may become pregnant, regardless of their gender identification.

REPRODUCTIVE JUSTICE Reproductive justice is an intersectional theory born from the experiences of women of color. The term was coined in 1994 by African American women after the International Conference on Population and Development in Cairo, Egypt, and is based on the understanding that the impacts of race, class, gender, and sexual identity oppressions can not be untangled from each other. Reproductive justice articulates an affirmative role for government in supporting a woman's self-determination in her own reproductive destiny and asserts that her ability to access a "choice" is directly linked to the conditions in her community.

UNMEDICATED VAGINAL BIRTH *or* ***"NATURAL" BIRTH*** This occurs when no medications are used during labor, and the baby is delivered through the vaginal canal. Unmedicated vaginal birth has popularly been called "natural" birth in many doula and birthing communities. Some birth justice activists are now trying to move away from that term, as it may imply that "natural" is better than surgical, and can be a shaming agent for women who have interventions such as C-sections.

The Rise of Reproductive Justice and the Doula Project:
A (Very) Brief Timeline

1966 Reverend Howard Moody cofounds the Clergy Consultation Service—a national network of Protestant and Jewish clergy who helped women find safe, confidential, and compassionate abortions—out of Judson Memorial Church on lower Fifth Avenue in Manhattan.

1969 Anthropologist Dana Raphael uses the term "doula" in a study related to birth outcomes. Many people trained in massage, physical therapy, midwifery, and other fields begin to attend births regularly; among them is Penny Simkin, who will later popularize the term among birth advocates with her written guidelines and suggestions.

The Jane Collective, a group of feminists (none of whom are medical professionals), begins performing safe, affordable abortions in homes and apartments in Chicago as a response to the costs as well as the number of injuries and deaths due to unsafe procedures performed illegally—and thus with no regulation.

1970 Abortion becomes legal in four states—Hawaii, New York, Washington, and Alaska—as well as DC. The original *Our Bodies, Ourselves* (then titled *Women and Their Bodies*) is published, putting women's health in a new feminist political and social context.

January 22, 1973 *Roe v. Wade* means that abortion is legal in all fifty states and concretizes pregnancy "trimesters."

1970s Holistically minded feminist women's health clinics such as Preterm in Cleveland, Choices in Memphis, CHOICES in Queens, and the Feminist Women's Health Centers (in California and Atlanta, among others) incorporate patient support into the fabric of their clinic structure. These roles, sometimes known as "patient supporters" or "hand holders," are often performed by paid clinic staff members and speak to how these clinics prioritize compassionate patient service as part of the abortion experience. Studies that show the benefits of having professional labor support during birth emerge. These improvements include better pain management, shorter labors, lower use of epidural anesthesia, fewer labor inductions, and fewer C-sections.

1975 George Tiller takes the helm of the Women's Health Care Services in Wichita, Kansas, one of three centers in the country that provide abortions past twenty-four weeks. Initially, Tiller intended to be a dermatologist, but after seeing a woman die from an illegal procedure, he decided to follow in the footsteps of his father, an abortion provider.

1976 Congress passes the Hyde Amendment, which makes it illegal to use federal funding to pay for abortions (states may allocate funds as they wish). Because abortion technically remains "legal" and Hyde mainly affects low-income people who use Medicaid, the limitations it imposes on abortion access are accepted. For many women, the Hyde Amendment negates the access created by *Roe v. Wade*.

1978 Ina May Gaskin's *Spiritual Midwifery* is published, a beacon of natural childbirth. Doulas and midwives will quote from, love, and use this book for generations to come.

1989 Penny Simkin publishes *The Birth Partner*, the "gold standard" of doula care in the years to come.

1992 The first birth-doula certifying organization, Doulas of North America (DONA), is founded, soon followed by others. Further restrictions to abortion are codified in *Planned Parenthood v. Casey*.

1994 In September the Cairo International Conference on Population and Development redefines reproductive health as a human right. African American women at the conference coin the phrase "reproductive justice" to challenge the notion that all women have enough access to resources to make reproductive "choices."

1997 SisterSong, a woman-of-color led collective emphasizing a holistic model of reproductive healthcare and access, forms. SisterSong's vision looks beyond abortion access and contraception—a narrative that some felt were akin to population control. People come together from across the divide of pro-choice and antiabortion to offer an intersectional political framework. The group labels their work "reproductive justice."

1999 The Ryan Program Fellowship in Reproductive Choice and Family Planning is founded to increase training in abortion procedures at medical schools and residency programs.

2000 Medical abortion—RU486 or mifepristone—becomes legal in the US.

2003 The Partial-Birth Abortion Ban is passed, criminalizing doctors who perform "intact" dilation and evacuation procedures—the safest method of abortion for pregnancies that are past twenty weeks' gestation. This has a dramatic impact on the way that providers are trained to do the procedure, as well as on access for patients to obtain these procedures.

2006 Ann Fessler's *The Girls Who Went Away* is published and addresses mid-twentieth-century adoption practices based on oral histories with birth mothers. The book is a bestseller and a revelation, shedding new light on the birth mother experience.

2007 The National Advocates for Pregnant Women Summit, Civil Liberties and Public Policy (CLPP) Conference, and New York City Birth Coalition Summit catalyze the Doula Project founders (Mary, Lauren, Pérez) to envision our program, which we come to call the "Abortion Doula Project."

2008 After the Abortion Doula Project formally partners with the City Hospital Reproductive Choices Service, Spence-Chapin—a pro-choice adoption agency—and the Adoption Access Network, we hold our first national training with a group in Atlanta, Georgia. We change our name to the Doula Project and use the phrase "Supporting people throughout the spectrum of pregnancy outcomes" on our informational postcards. We call ourselves "full-spectrum doulas," and the term takes off. *The Business of Being Born*, released as a response to a national C-section rate that is at or above 30 percent of all births, further emboldens us.

2009 George Tiller is assassinated by an antiabortion activist in May; communities involved in reproductive healthcare and justice mourn. There remain four other clinics in the country that perform abortions past the second trimester.

2010 We begin our partnership with Planned Parenthood of New York City in their Brooklyn clinic in May, thanks to doula/LC member Jini Tanenhaus, and establish our birth-doula service for low-income clients. In the fall, an influx of antichoice congress members and governors are elected, beginning a multiyear trend that has devastating impact on women's and LGBTQ rights across the country. We partner with CHOICES, a local Queens clinic that sees a high volume of patients.

2011 We have trained eighty doulas. Planned Parenthood conducts a small "Acceptability and Feasibility" study of our volunteer model, afterwhich we partner with the Bronx Planned Parenthood.

2012 We have trained 110 doulas. City Hospital closes for several months due to Hurricane Sandy on October 30. The City Hospital Reproductive Choices Service moves to Bushwick Hospital during this time.

2013 The Doula Project has worked with over twenty thousand clients and trained over a dozen doula groups nationally. After doing four years of stillbirth inductions at City Hospital, we begin working with their birth program to provide doula support on labor and delivery.

2014 In addition to training another thirty-five new doulas, we partner with the Bronx Defenders, assisting people who are at risk for losing their children.

2015 In the summer, the antichoice movement releases egregious video footage to sabotage Planned Parenthood. This further exacerbates the Republican attack on abortion and puts Planned Parenthood at risk of losing nationwide funding. A deadly shooting at a Colorado Springs Planned Parenthood clinic in December further highlights the dire divide between the pro-choice and antichoice movement.

2016 In March, the Doula Project begins paying stipends to all doulas, including those attending abortions. The Supreme Court hands down *Whole Woman's Health v. Hellerstedt*, overturning nuisance laws that had threatened to shut down many clinics. The Doula Project recruits and trains another group of abortion doulas, bringing our total number trained to more than two hundred in New York City alone and has educated more than a dozen groups of activists, doulas, and clinicians nationwide.

Acknowledgments

Writing this book was an emotional journey through time. As this book is being released, we are celebrating nearly a decade of serving clients as full-spectrum doulas. We feel privileged to have had the opportunity to reflect on the work of the Doula Project in such an in-depth and profound way. We have so many people who supported us, inspired us, and worked alongside us as we wrote this book.

First we want to thank the Doula Project members, providers, and clients who spent hours and hours with us sharing your stories. Your honesty, your self-awareness, your ability to take your stories to sad or scary or provocative places, and, most of all, your trust in us gives this book its strength and power. The way you engage as doulas and human beings truly shaped the way this book was written. A million thanks to Vicki Bloom, Kat Broadway, Miriam Cremer, Poonam Dreyfus-Pai, Kale Edmiston, Kiya Freeman, Kira Laffe, Mallory Mahoney, Amita Murthy, Bri Tristan, Symone New, Miriam Zoila Pérez, Annie

Robinson, Danika Severino Wynn, Whitney Tucker, and Treasure Walker. Thank you also to the clients we could not reach and to those contributors who wish to remain unnamed.

We also want to thank our movement allies and the other doula organizations who provided invaluable historical and philosophical contributions to this book during one-on-one interviews. Thank you to Aspen Baker, Nafeesa Dawoodbhoy, Marci Leiber, Laura Kaplan, Marlene Gerber Fried, Melissa Madera, Grayson Morris, Lynn Paltrow, Janna Slack, Sarah Whedon, Amy Silverman (who coined "ambiguous loss") and the many other colleagues and supporters we have referenced throughout the book. Thank you to Ann Fessler who gave us invaluable advice on how to conduct oral histories in responsible and effective ways. Special thanks to Aimee Thorne-Thomsen, who served as reader and advisor to the book, in addition to her role of lifelong mentor and dear friend. Thank you also to Renee Bracey Sherman for serving as reader and thought contributor.

Thank you to Loretta Ross for writing an amazing foreword and for believing in our work and in this book. Thank you to Dr. Willie Parker for the afterword of our dreams.

Thank you to our editor Jennifer Baumgardner, who approached us to write this book and coached us throughout the process. Your confidence in us—and your expertise—is the reason this book exists at all. We are so proud to be part of the legendary Feminist Press!

Mary would like to give thanks to her mom Peggy Dawson for a lifetime of wisdom and guidance, and her siblings, Mike and Mallory, for being her constant sidekicks and soul mates. She gives special thanks to her dad, Jack Mahoney, for his brilliant copyediting skills, and to her partner, Brendan Bliss, for not only providing key structural edits but helping her rethink entire sections of the book. Thank you to Katrina Cass for being a wonderful thought partner and sponsoring many writing retreats, to Meredith Dreiman for everything since seventh grade, and to Ian Daniel for helping her remember why she became a doula in the first place.

Lauren would like to personally thank her parents, Bill and Sandy Mitchell, and her sisters, Lisa and Jessica, for all of their support. She gives special thanks to Kale Edmiston, who not only provided an incredible oral history but also made sure she was fed, watered, and cared for throughout the writing of this book. Thanks to Chelsea Miller (and Finch, Shephard, and Kevin) for being a veritable fountain of love at all times, to her work-wife Melissa Castro, her City Hospital family with whom she shares an irreplaceable bond, and to her Vanderbilt mentors and colleagues, who have cheered her on and pushed her to become a better writer.

Finally, thank you to the Doula Project itself—the Leadership Circle, Board of Directors, and current and former doulas—for their support during the writing of this book. Special thanks to current and former project leaders who haven't already been mentioned: Nicole Clark, Risa Cromer, Laura Duncan, Cecilia Duran, Ilana Dzuba, Andie Gersh, Kristin Giroux, Riley Ingram, Lily Jordahl, Maura Larkin,

Taja Lindley, Sarah McCarry, Mick Moran, Wendy Nguyen, Lola Pellegrino, Kathleen Reutter, Julia Rothschild, Alanah Roy, Jini Tanenhaus, El Tarver, Lucy Trainor, and Kyle Vereyken.

Thanks to our partners and clinics and everyone who has supported the Doula Project for the past decade.

The **Feminist Press** is a nonprofit educational organization founded to amplify feminist voices. FP publishes classic and new writing from around the world, creates cutting-edge programs, and elevates silenced and marginalized voices in order to support personal transformation and social justice for all people.

See our complete list of books at
feministpress.org

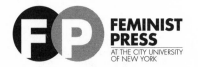

31901060062520